Bedside Manner

A Practical Guide To Interacting With Patients

David R. Coleman, MPAS, PA-C

Publication Consultants Since 1978

PO Box 221974 Anchorage, Alaska 99522-1974
books@publicationconsultants.com—www.publicationconsultants.com

ISBN 978-1-59433-061-2
eBook ISBN 978-1-59433-199-2

Library of Congress Catalog Card Number: 2007928052

—First Edition—

Chapter illustrations by Robert Ferrin Gilmore

Manufactured in the United States of America.

Dedication

To my lovely wife, Karen,
who is every bit my better half;
and our two sons, Brian and Nathan.
You bring my heart great joy.

Contents

Acknowledgments

I owe a tremendous debt of gratitude to those who have taken the time to educate me. Their patience and understanding guided me through many challenges. My parents, Ed and Julie Coleman, inspired me to maintain an insatiable appetite for learning. My teachers, formal and informal, taught me not only technical skills and principles, but by example, showed me how to be a better person. Through daily interaction with my supervising physicians, co-workers, friends, and patients, I began to understand the art of medicine more completely. This dynamic continues today. Thank you all from the bottom of my heart.

Foreword

The year prior to completing this book, I worked as a locums provider in Washington State, Oklahoma, and Alaska. That experience showed me different medical process environments. Though all desired satisfactory patient outcomes while maximizing healthcare resources, some facilities built that concept into their plans. Others actually had regulations that impeded such results. These areas of friction easily affected the demeanor of the staff and providers. Not that good bedside manner was absent in such places, just more elusive.

As the book explains, bedside manner is more than just the interaction between a provider and his patient. Everyone and everything related to a given facility has an impact on the overall patient experience. If that is not taken into consideration, the interaction is doomed from the start. We hope that the frustrations placed on our staff through poor processes never show to the patient. But that is just not the case. Staff frustrations easily spill over into patient interactions.

My desire is that this book will help healthcare professionals across the globe look at bedside manner in a different light in order to give it the best chance of success. Too often the fault for a bad patient experience is placed at the feet of the provider. Remember that bedside manner is not a solo, but a symphony. We all play a part and share in the results. Thank you for allowing me, through this book, to participate in yours.

Chapter One

What is Bedside Manner?

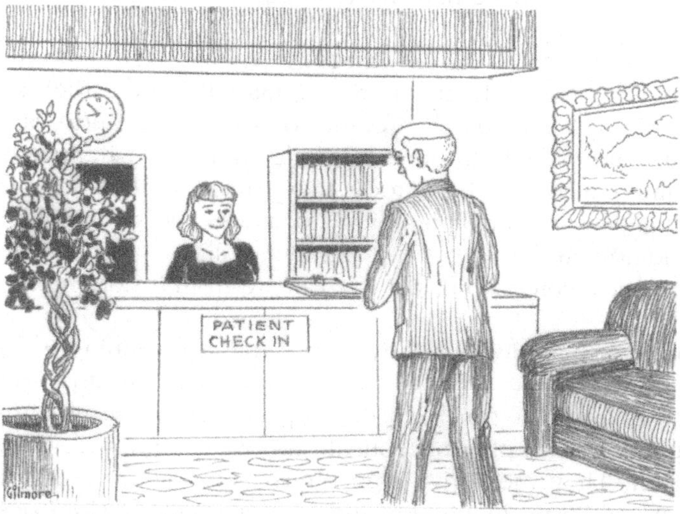

In February 2002, the British press announced that a formal course was being developed to help doctors improve their communication skills. This was inspired by Cancer Research UK.[1] Inadequacies were commonplace when doctors were communicating bad news to patients and their families. So a three-day course was created to enhance physician communication skills in dealing with such issues.

That same year, the United States National Board of Medical Examiners announced they had developed a "clinical skills assessment" test to evaluate the communication skills of physicians in America. The test would be six hours long and place medical students with actors posing as patients. The students would then be evaluated on how they handled approximately 10-12 fifteen minute sessions.[2]

Throughout the world, governments are looking at how their

doctors communicate with patients. This goes above their ability to diagnose and treat illnesses and injuries. Instead, it relates more to their ability to care. Though medical schools generally produce competent healthcare providers, compassion remains a difficult subject to instill and retain. No one educational system has shown itself to be more effective than the other in solving this shortcoming.

History

The term "bedside manner" originated from earlier times when physicians used to come to your house and evaluate you from your bedside using little more than their clinical acumen and some basic tools they carried in their bag. They focused more on their ability to assess the overall human condition and less on the particular illness within. Family dynamics were also easier to evaluate from inside the home.

Today, a majority of a physician's medical training is spent learning disease processes and appropriate lab and special studies available for diagnostic support. They learn treatment regimens and pharmaceutical options to improve patient health. They memorize algorithms in order to identify and treat conditions in a timely and efficient manner. Compassion and caring has been placed on the "learn as you go" shelf.

Present Contrast

But if physicians were miraculously granted the ability to communicate with all of the patients in their practice, would that create perfect "bedside manner?" In the old days of house calls, it might. But in today's society, bedside manner takes on a whole new meaning. Now patients come to the healthcare provider's clinic or "home." They observe our staff or "family" dynamics and interact on our terms. They're taken from what they know as comfortable and placed into our "sterile" foreign environments.

Some of the old social norms visitors used to expect from hosts are lost when they visit our clinic. Though they have an appointment and are expected, instead of being made comfortable and treated as a guest of the facility, they are often greeted in typical soup-line fashion and instructed to promptly begin filling out forms requesting a myriad of personal information. They're asked to wait for long periods of time in small waiting rooms with other individuals who they do not know.

Once back in the deeper chambers of our clinic, they're required to get out of their comfortable clothes and put on outfits they neither requested nor desire. Then they're subjected to needle sticks, weight evaluations, and told to provide samples of items they rather not keep. In some situations, patients are then asked to position themselves in a manner that exposes areas of their body reserved for the most intimate of companions. It's about this time that they're greeted by the doctor.

Now no one expects a clinic to truly act as a home, but as the saying goes, "hope springs eternal." In the above example, the doctor has just entered the room, yet the patient had more than enough opportunity to evaluate the "bedside manner" of this clinic and indirectly, of the physician. If this were indeed a home setting, it would be easy to see how someone could get very offended being handled so carelessly. Yet it remains a common occurrence done in the name of expedience.

Evaluation

This clinic failed to provide a pleasurable experience. They didn't show much interest or care for the concerns of the patient. They had an unwavering system to support and no time for such luxuries as common courtesy. Getting patients through the system became more important than actually taking care of them. By the time the patient interacted with the doctor, the groundwork for dissatisfaction had already been laid.

The overall experience might at best be viewed as tolerable if the provider is an excellent communicator. Or perhaps the patient might be insightful enough to distinguish between the bedside manner of the clinic and that of the doctor. Would that benefit the doctor? Not really, since the doctor is ultimately in charge of all clinic happenings and the experience would most likely be repeated at each visit. And often the provider is too busy to even realize what sort of presentation his or her clinic is showing the patient.

Unfortunately, whether by desire or design, all providers feel varying degrees of time constraints throughout their day. Most clinics keep a routine pace where patients are fed into the system at fifteen minute intervals. In specialty clinics, this is almost workable, since patients usually have similar symptoms and complaints. In family practice or other general medicine clinics, fifteen minutes to talk to the patient, perform an exam, diagnose a condition, plan a course of action, and explain it to the patient becomes a daunting challenge. Where one patient might complain of a rash, the next might describe a cardiac condition or rectal bleeding that would require a much greater work-up. To take more time with one patient then affects the next. In no time at all, we providers find ourselves working through lunch and staying after hours to finish our schedules.

The finer points of bedside manner are eventually pushed aside in the perpetual desire to streamline activities. Because it's far more expedient to be undressed and ready for the exam at the start, it's not uncommon for many doctors to have their patients in exam gowns and/or examination position prior to being greeted. Some even explain their findings and finish the meeting without the patient even getting up or getting dressed. It's not too hard for doctors to eventually become cynical over the requirements of the job. Some even pride themselves on their ability to minimize their patient interaction time. One doctor, prior to entering a room to perform an annual pap exam actually told me, "I'll be in and out of there in thirty seconds. Time me."

Though that might seem a bit harsh, think of the pace through a non-medical perspective. Suppose you were required to attend a meeting. In it, you would have to be both the leader and the secretary. You would be expected to interact with the group, evaluate any information presented, decide frequently on life and death issues and act on a plan for success, get "buy-in" from the rest of the group and create legal documentation of the entire event all within fifteen minutes. Now suppose you had to meet with different groups and be responsible for similar activities every fifteen minutes for eight hours a day, five days a week. So is the daily life of a healthcare provider. Stress and fatigue can quickly take their toll. The system encourages brevity and impersonal interaction.

As the healthcare provider, responsibility for the overall experience the patient has is thought to rest with you. Bedside manner is felt to be completely your domain. But this is really not the case. The concept of beside manner belongs to all who interact with the patient. From the front desk person who initially takes the appointment call all the way to the doctor who treats the patient. Everyone plays a part in the experience the patient walks away with. The Horizon Group noted this when, in 1997, they identified four separate areas that contribute to patient satisfaction in a clinic environment. In their Family Practice survey, they found that not only the physicians, but the front office staff, the ambience of the practice facility, and the clinical support staff all played key roles in patient satisfaction.[3]

Think of it in a personal manner. Before we go out our doors, we clean ourselves up, put on our chosen deodorant and perfume (or cologne), select what we feel is the right outfit to highlight our positive attributes (something clean and pressed, no doubt), insure our hair style is perfect, and then head out into our daily activities. Those we interact with might look at us and say, "What a pleasant person." They probably didn't take time to examine every nuance of our presentation. They just subconsciously took in all of the individual components we previously addressed and came to an overall conclusion.

Now suppose something was not "normal" in your presentation. If in a business office, one day you wore sweatpants instead of the usual attire. Even though you might act exactly the same as before, people would come to different conclusions about you. They might assume you're flawed in some way. Or maybe if you had buttoned your shirt or blouse off by one button all the way down that might garner more attention throughout the day than any other correct thing you did. A more subtle example seen every day is the friend who

> ℞ IF YOU KNEW THAT INCREASED ATTENTION TO SOME DETAIL WOULD IMPROVE CUSTOMER LOYALTY, HOW MUCH MORE ATTENTION WOULD YOU BE WILLING TO FOCUS ON IT?

presents with a piece of food stuck in their teeth. It doesn't take long to become totally distracted by the error.

Medical bedside manner works in much the same way. If everything is at its best, the provider is allowed to add the finishing touches and make the overall experience more enjoyable. If, however, the staff or environment is found to be lacking in some way, the provider may not be able to recover the encounter. All aspects of the clinic must work together to present a total experience.

This total experience concept is not unique to the medical field. In his book, *Inside the Magic Kingdom–Seven Keys to Disney's Success,* Tom Connellan highlighted the tremendous detailing that the Disney Corporation performs each day in order to create the perfect vacation experience for their guests. Some are not even seen by the average guest, but are instead purely for the benefit of the employees. It allows them to see how intricate the balance of detail plays on everything they do. Even calling the employees "cast members" implies maintaining a "stage presence" mentality in their workdays.

"...If you knew that increased attention to some detail would improve customer loyalty, how much more attention would you be willing to focus on it?"[(4)] This type of question is rarely pursued in patient interactions. Yet it should be considered with every staff member who comes in verbal, visual, or physical contact with a patient. How they look, sound and act is a direct reflection on how patients perceive you think and care about them. Therefore, it's important to examine the entire facility presentation from the patient's point of view. How does the

facility look? Is it clean? Does it look run-down or unkempt? Are there things to keep patients occupied while they wait for their appointment? Have basic needs of patients been met?

What about the staff? Do they all match or at least have on nice clothes or do they all look like they just came out of a high school classroom? Are they speaking respectfully to patients or in a condescending manner? In what ways can each of these issues be improved? Are we improving to be the best we can for our patients or just to be better than our local competition?

Bedside manner should be a concept owned by all and not just the provider. Its success or failure rests in the hands of everyone who interacts with the patient: Absolutely everyone! Failure in one area easily negates any other successes. As the saying goes, "You never get a second chance to make a first impression." Disney's tactics were thought of as extreme back in his early days, but the outcome speaks for itself. Had he not been so meticulous, his company might have turned out to be just another amusement park. Instead, Disney remains the cherished household name it's been for decades.

The fantasy needs to be complete in order to maintain its allure for everyone. To see the building facades and framework behind the scenes would ruin the overall effect. To watch the cast-members play gleefully with patrons and then hang around listlessly in a visible smoking section would also be detrimental to the visual panorama being performed on-site. Your bedside manner should be held in the same regard. From the time your patient begins their interaction until it ends, they reside in the world you've created for them.

To that end, make sure your entire staff is familiar with the basics of interpersonal communication as well as the layout and procedures of the clinic. The front office personnel will be the most likely first-responders to patient questions. They need to know how to properly answer basic clinical questions and how to get answers for the more technical issues. Failure to invest in their training is to risk the clinic's initial presentation as ignorant and uncaring.

> **℞ The Waiter Rule**
>
> An accurate representation of your true character is found in the way you treat a servant.

The well-being of others is a very familiar concept to providers. But should that only extend to our patients? Is it only because they're paying us that we should choose to show kindness? If so, that's a sad commentary on our character. To show kindness to a patient in one breath and then belittle a staff member in the next shows insincerity to all witnesses. Yet, this happens frequently throughout the nation's clinics, wards, and operating rooms. Not only for providers, but many in authority tend to take this approach. As Lord Acton once said, "Power tends to corrupt and absolute power corrupts absolutely." The lay public has a term called *The Waiter Rule* which says that the way one treats servants is a more accurate representation of their character.

Sharon the ER nurse set up a suture tray for Dr. P in room 7 as requested. The patient, a 42 year old mother of two, had suffered a small scalp laceration earlier. He saw her when she first came in and had her wound cleaned. He seemed very knowledgeable about her condition and his expertise helped allay her fears. It was a busy night, so he excused himself to check on some other patients while things were being prepared. Upon his return, he put on sterile gloves and was sitting down to stitch her up when he noticed the tray was missing a needle holder for his suture. Without warning, he threw the instrument tray across the room and exclaimed to Sharon, "Are you thinking at all tonight? This set-up is incomplete. Now get me a complete tray and don't call me back until its ready!" With that, he took off his gloves and stormed out of the room.

Dr. P had started out doing well for his patient, but the shallowness of his character quickly surfaced when interacting with his staff. To show compassion in one moment and outright aggression the next only exhibits insincerity to all. Dr. P's attempt at bedside manner was nullified through his actions with his nurse. And it made Sharon's credibility suspect as well.

Tensions are usually heightened in emergent situations and it's easy to forgo good bedside manner and blame it on expedience. With all the chaos of the average emergency room occurring 24 hours a day, it seems natural to yell just to be heard above the roar. But without good, calm interaction, quality care is more likely to be hindered. The patient's view is usually limited to what's in front of their face and watching people scream around them is counter-productive. Simple explanations and a relaxed manner are ideal when talking to or around a patient. "One of our nurses is going to start an IV in your left arm, so you'll feel her checking your arm for a vein. After that, you'll feel a little poke when she puts the IV in, but she'll warn you before she does it." It's hard to take their feelings into consideration during stressful times, but realize patients are observing very unfamiliar activities and feeling varying degrees of pain and anxiety. Helping them cope will go a long way to keeping them calm and emotionally healthy.

> *Dr. F was a well known general surgeon who shared trauma on-call responsibilities with several other surgeons in his group. The ER personnel always dreaded when he was on-call because he was quick to yell and verbally abuse staff members whenever he was called in. Everybody felt extra stress beyond just taking care of the critical patient. "Code" situations seemed more disorganized and hectic. Since things always ran smoother when his partners were there and no other surgeon acted that way, it was easy to see to all around him that he really was more insecure with himself than in the staff, but that was his way of handling it.*

We're quick to abuse staff, especially in medicine. Mistakes, though considered learning opportunities elsewhere, are not allowed in the medical arena. Many are sacrificed so that others may remain unscathed. A nurse practitioner friend of mine told me she left the nursing career for just such a reason. "The nursing field is cannibalistic. They eat their own. The chief nurse eats the charge nurses. The charge nurses eat the staff nurses. The staff nurses eat the staff." Unfortunately, this behavior can be seen in other professions as well.

The practice of belittling makes for poor self-esteem among the staff and poor performance in their work. Such situations over time tend to anesthetize people from the caring aspect of their activities and focus them only on the mechanics of their duties. This change of heart is palpable by all who come in contact with it and serves as the underlying foundation for many patient complaints. But are the patients we currently care for our only customers?

> *While doing rounds on the surgical ward, Dr. R, a first year resident, got into a discussion with some of the staff. It was lighthearted and some benign jokes were made about the habits of some of the patients recovering there. Dr. H, the attending with him, took him aside. "Be careful about using patients as a source of your jokes." "Oh, don't worry," Dr. R. said. "No patients were around." Dr. H stepped in close. "Not only is it generally inappropriate, but your staff member today could be your patient tomorrow. If that happens, they'll remember how you treated past patients and their information. That could mean the difference between them coming to see you or your competition. Be compassionate and respectful in all situations."*

From the department store clerk to the grocery store bagger, everyone is a potential patient. Your interaction with them is not so much a testimony of who they are as it is who you are. If you are only willing to show kindness to those who can afford it or to those who first show it to you, insincerity and distrust will be your presentation. As a professional, you represent yourself 24 hours a day; not just during working hours. True bedside manner needs to be with you wherever you go. Only then will it become internalized and flow naturally to others.

Chapter Two
Caring 101

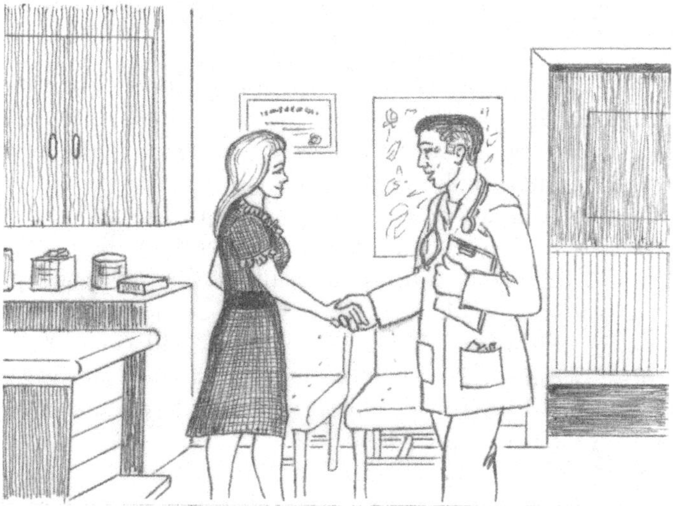

"I waited for the doctor almost an hour before they put me in the exam room and I waited there another 30 minutes before he finally came in. He was in a hurry and only stayed about 30 seconds before he rushed out the door. I didn't even get a chance to ask any questions."

In today's microwave society, not everything is viewed better when it's done faster. Where healthcare is concerned, patients prefer a little more personal one-on-one time instead of assembly-line medicine. They want to know more about what's happening to them. Not so much the technical details, but the overall basics of their condition. They prefer we be fast with others so we can be on time with them and available for all of their questions. Patients desire to have access to their providers any time they deem necessary for as long as possible.

As providers, we're trained to question everything. We're taught that patients always have two agendas; the one they're telling you about and the one they're not. They rarely exhibit purely noble intentions. At times, they're out for money (through litigation), drug-seeking, or out for some satisfaction through manipulation. Sometimes they're just not able to explain themselves very well, which forces you to be even more diligent about getting the right information to make the correct diagnosis.

Having a successful interaction quickly becomes a great challenge. Because prices per visit are spartan (and sometimes only partially paid), we're forced to see more patients in less time in order to make ends meet. This makes us either ask fewer questions at each visit or speak quickly and not allow for further concerns. Patients feel rushed in their appointment and unloved. In no time at all we change from quality care givers to quantity care givers in order to meet the daily demands of the job. Though quality is still on our minds, it's now positioned farther back in our algorithm. For some providers, rushing through their schedule becomes an all too common occurrence.

In our attempt to be prompt, we've forgotten to care about our patients. I was going to say that caring is a basic obligation in our profession, but that's incorrect. Nowhere in the Hippocratic Oath does it say we're required to care for patients. It says that we're required to treat them. Many, unfortunately, take that loop-hole to heart and mistake treatment for caring. Patients, however, still consider caring an integral component of the overall treatment process. Like water for flowers, the act of caring is essential for maintaining a healthy patient.

While working in a busy emergency room one night, a patient started our encounter with, "I hope you're not one of those mean doctors." Though I'd heard that statement before, for some reason it seemed more poignant that night. It's a sad commentary on the overall state of medicine for patients to worry so. The thought that "mean doctors" are still so common as to be an open concern was disheartening. Considering the nature of the profession, why would anybody choose to be mean?

Did she label her previous provider "mean" merely because he failed to give in to her desires? Or are there doctors and other healthcare professionals who truly don't play well with others? As healthcare providers, we should strive to show caring and compassion in all our activities. Whether it's treating someone in need or denying an unhealthy request, the patient should leave knowing they interacted with a friend and their best interests were the basis for our actions.

So how does one show they care and yet avoid negatively impacting other appointments? Is there enough time in the day to allow for quality interaction for all? Does the addition of "caring" require some subtraction in "treating?" Since there's no ICD-9 code for caring, is it really worth the effort? I once quoted a phrase I heard in childhood to one of my co-workers; "Kindness doesn't cost extra." To my amazement, the reply came back, "Yeah? Well, it doesn't pay extra either." He failed to see that people don't appreciate being herded indiscriminately through a system like cattle. They prefer to be treated with kindness and compassion, and are willing to travel to find it.

The concept of caring can be broken down into one simple phrase…the golden rule; "Do unto others as you would have them do unto you." It doesn't take much effort at all on our part to provide great emotional benefit for the patient. Practically speaking, here are several tips that I've found to be invaluable in creating a positive environment. They come from years of personal experience and recommendations from many well-respected colleagues.

Pre-Visit Preparation

Before we utter a word, let's first consider out attire. Like decorations adorning the walls in our house, our dress and appearance create a statement about us. Are we relaxed or stuffy? Are we serious or comical? Have we taken time to address the basics, such as our clothes being clean and pressed? Even simpler, does our clothes match?

How about the lab coat? This is an item with a great deal of controversy. From region to region, state to state, town to town, even provider to provider. We all have opinions about whether or not a lab coat is necessary. It definitely has functional use. Pockets enough to keep several quick references, a PDA, a stethoscope, and a prescription pad at the ready. It can also serve to identify providers from a distance and create a sense of uniformity among them. Embroidered names are easily readable from afar.

On the negative side; a lab coat can inspire a degree of "white-coat syndrome." In the average clinical setting this may be an infrequent occurrence and of no significant concern. But where the patient population is primarily psychiatric, the lab coat could be an obstacle to more effective communication. In warmer climates, it might be an uncomfortably hot addition to one's attire. Ease of movement could also be impaired with their use. And in surgical situations where coats are donned and doffed frequently, leaving your lab coat in forgotten locations would pose a daily concern.

The clothes you choose to wear to work may also determine the need for a lab coat. If jeans are comfortable to you yet a more professional air at work is desired, the lab coat may solve your problem. If wearing a suit comes naturally to you, the lab coat may be an unnecessary addition. Some choose to dress "down" so as not to make their patients feel uncomfortable with their own appearance. Whatever the choice regarding dress and lab coat use, it should be made after careful consideration of local norms and expectations.

The Encounter

When you enter an exam room, introduce yourself to everyone in the room, not just the patient. Though the patient is the reason for the appointment, everyone in the room should have an opportunity to make eye contact with you and shake your hand. Avoiding individuals in a small group setting, whether it be an exam room or a party, makes them feel unappreciated. Without introductions to establish formal channels of communication, people are less apt to volunteer potentially important information.

After your introductions, be sure to sit down. Standing makes it seem like you're about to leave the room and go to a more important meeting. It creates an undo sense of anxiety. It also places your head above all others. By sitting, you present less of a threatening appearance and show a willingness to stay awhile.

There should be enough seats available for you and the patient plus one or two additional guests. If the patient has taken your rolling chair but there are enough seats still for all, invite him or her to sit on the exam table. "To better help identify all of the players, why don't you come sit up here and I'll take that seat," you might say. If readjusting appears too problematic, take whatever seat is available, even if it's only the exam table. Adjustment can be made when you get to performing the exam.

The History

When acquiring a history, make your patient feel like they're having a comfortable exchange of information between two old friends instead of an interrogation. A common problem for new providers is to be so concerned about the questions they need answered, they forget they're in the midst of a conversation. Answers are acknowledged only long enough to jot them down. Basic rapport is rarely attempted. Other than being medically focused, the interaction should feel natural.

Effective communication requires a sender, the transmission, and a receiver. Though we're quick to send transmissions to the patient, we often fail to interact with information we receive. Without responding appropriately to the patient's answers, we appear to be uninterested and uncaring. Don't be afraid to base future questions on current answers.

An integral part of any "normal" interaction is eye contact. When friends get together to talk, they pay attention to each other and do their best to ignore extraneous distractions. As providers, we should also do our best to focus on our patients. Every person we speak to should be extended the courtesy of good eye contact throughout the interaction. Avoid asking questions and then looking down into the chart or into a computer monitor during the answer.

Start by asking an open-ended question, such as, "So, what brings you here today?" It's not uncommon for patients to have a chief complaint different from the one given to other staff members. By using an open-ended approach, it allows them, in their own words, to guide you directly to their concerns.

Once your initial question is asked, allow the patient time to answer. A 1999 article in JAMA found that the average patient in the United States is given only 22 seconds to make their initial statement before being interrupted by the provider.[5] Providers felt the need to interrupt in order to keep the patients on task. In 2002, Langewitz et al evaluated 335 patients to see what would happen if patients were allowed to complete their introductory comments uninterrupted. They found that almost 80% of patients finished all they had to say in 2 minutes or less before turning the conversation back over to the doctor. These patients, by the way, were from a tertiary referral center where complex histories were common.[6]

When someone feels the need to vent or "get this off my chest," interrupting them only impairs communication. Most people, afraid they might forget their issues, focus mainly on their thoughts and are not ready to hear input from anyone else. Only by allowing them to voice their concerns at the start will their minds be open to interaction. By allowing them to voice their concerns uninterrupted, improvements have been noted in patient satisfaction and information gathering without an extension of visit time.[7]

Show yourself through non-verbal cues to be "open" to the patient/group interaction. Maintain good eye contact with everyone. If notes are needed during the visit, make them brief and be sure to look up frequently and acknowledge the speaker. Try not to hide behind obstructions such as a desk or the chart. Don't use such non-verbal distractors as crossed legs or arms.

Leave your biases at the door. Personal information is entrusted to you in order to help you make an accurate diagnosis. This type of interaction is valuable and should be safeguarded. Exhibiting outward signs of disgust or outrage does nothing to help you gather the information you need. Instead it increases your risk of coming to the wrong conclusions and showing your ignorance.

> *Lisa was a 28 year old female who went to an oral surgeon's office for a pre-operative evaluation. She had impacted wisdom teeth and wanted them removed. During the evaluation, she informed him that her past surgical history included bilateral breast augmentations. His immediate verbal response was, "Oh, you're one of them." Though she had the reconstructive procedure several years back to repair her breast asymmetry, the oral surgeon assumed the only reason for the procedure was breast enhancement and judged her based on that. She never returned to him for the procedure.*

Empathetically query the patient on any necessary information. Don't let the familiarity with your questions make you sound disinterested or mechanical. Always ask them in an honest and caring manner. You'll quickly find that the more caring you act, the more caring you actually become.

Try to not get too distracted from the issue. I occasionally treat prisoners brought in from nearby facilities dressed in orange jumpsuits and shackles. Though my curiosity is greatly peaked each time they come in, unless it directly relates to their chief complaint, I never ask the reason for their incarceration. I instead resolve to treat them as openly and compassionately as the next patient.

Another common distractor is the patient who acts abnormal, whether being outright abusive or perhaps mentally challenged. They force us to focus more actively on their psychological issues and less on their physical complaints. This presents a very common snare for the average provider. While still in training years ago, a schizophrenic patient with some abdominal complaints came to the internal medicine clinic for an evaluation. The staff was quick to point out that she was a frequent flyer and "don't worry about her. It's all in her head." The internist I was working with said something that has since served me well to this day. "Dave, always remember; mentally ill patients get sick, too. The fact that she has a psychiatric condition hasn't answered the question of whether or not she's physically ill." Mentally unstable, belligerent, drug-seeking, or unkempt. Regardless of what others call the patient, the overriding question should always be, "Yes, but are they sick?"

Remember that patients are made up of more than just a collection of chief complaints. They all have loved ones, hobbies, desires, and interests that impact their daily lives. Frequently, some of this information is expressed during a visit. Finding items of common interest are invaluable when initially trying to establish rapport. Perhaps you both do needlecrafts. Or maybe you're both into sports. It might even relate to common locations traveled. Whatever it is, finding a common bond allows you to honestly engage in mutually stimulating *non-medical* conversation during your exam.

Regardless of whether or not it's an item of common interest, make a brief mention of some interesting non-medical item in your note. This will greatly aid your ability to connect at future visits. Discussions will become smoother since they'll feel more natural and less like a "sterile" environment. Conversations can feel more relaxed and less like a medical inquisition. Patients often respond positively when allowed to share a bit more than just their medical health.

I first learned this technique while working for a local surgeon. I would review his notes and noticed he quite frequently would add something to the bottom of his notes like, "Bill enjoys fly fishing and ties his own flies." When in the room with the patient he would casually comment on it during his exam. "So how's the fishing going?" "Catch anything interesting lately?" "Really? Did you use any special flies for that one?" It just flowed so naturally for him and the patients couldn't believe that he always seemed to remember specific things about them. They loved him for it.

Though this is an excellent way to show care for the patient as a whole, it must be tailored to fit into the ever pressing 15 minute time slot allotted. I use it best after I've acquired the information I need for the exam. Once I've written down my medically relevant concerns, I then put the chart away and go wash my hands before I examine my patient. While washing, I usually open the conversation up to the patient. By allowing some conversation to continue during the exam (except for where I really need quiet, such as listening for heart and lung sounds), patients tend to feel more comfortable and relaxed. Time also seems to suspend a bit as conversation continues. Since the information is not critical to their medical concerns, I don't usually write anything down. Conversation can just occur naturally. If anything relevant comes up, I can either remember it and write it down after the exam, or make a quick note in the chart and then return to the exam. The end of the exam creates a natural break and medical issues can once again be addressed.

When I first saw Katherine for her overactive bladder, she mentioned to me that she had two twin daughters in their junior year of high school. Amber wanted to be a pediatrician and Angela a gynecologist. They'd been receiving brochures from different universities and were unsure where they'd like to attend. I made a brief note about them and brought it up at our next visit. She was thrilled that I remembered to ask and glowed with pride as she informed me of their status. After one or two visits, it just came naturally that I recalled her children. No further notes about them were necessary.

Wrapping Up the Encounter

After the exam, be sure to tell the patient their diagnosis in a way they can understand. It's okay to use the correct term at first, but follow it with an explanation right after. "You have sinusitis. There are pockets behind your cheeks that are irritated and filling up with fluid and bacteria. I'm going to give you some medication to address the bacteria and the congestion." Patients who understand their malady are better equipped to support therapeutic interventions. Don't be afraid to use drawings or handouts to help them understand. Drug companies frequently print generic

> PATIENTS ARE MULTIFACETED. THERE'S MORE GOING ON THAN JUST THEIR DISEASE PROCESSES.

patient helps and are an excellent resource for such support.

Be honest in your interaction. If you feel uncomfortable providing a particular medication, be up front about it and explain your actions. Many times I had to tell someone I felt uncomfortable giving them narcotic medication because of their history of substance abuse, their current med use, or some other red-flag that gave me pause. But I let the patient know about it while in my presence. Truly hurting patients were usually thankful for whatever alternates I would recommend and drug-seekers would gripe a little more and then leave. Either way, I made them understand what I was going to do and why I was doing it.

If the system that I'm operating in forces my hand one way or another, I'm happy to let the patient know about that, too. Some formularies or policies require use of an older generic drug before a newer medication is prescribed. This is more commonly seen in government-run facilities. If that's the case, let the patient know a particular medicine is required to be used first. Patients appreciate honesty and usually understand organizational restrictions.

Get the patient involved in their own treatment. With the kind of medicine available today and the pressure for seeing as many patients as possible, it's very easy for providers to want to make a diagnosis, prescribe a medication and hustle the patient out the door. But that kind of mentality belittles the benefit of having a provider evaluation. The "take this pill and wait for your problems to go away" approach gives patients no responsibility in their treatment management. They have no buy-in. Anecdotally, treatment plans fare better when patient participation is used.

I try to live by the rule that if I only give the patient medication, I did them a disservice. I should also be able to advise them in some way to actively improve their chances of healing. Whether it be changing their diet or activities, or avoiding bad habits: Whatever they can do to improve their condition should be encouraged. Remember that patients are multifaceted. There's more going on than just their disease processes. To think that a given medication is the panacea for all their woes is a bit naive.

It was a difficult task early on in my medical career, since my personal experiences were few and school mainly focused on diagnosis and pharmaceutical intervention. But I was determined to make my encounters with the patient rewarding for all. Initially, I acquired a home remedy book an old physician wrote and started reading through the different conditions listed. Though I couldn't remember everything, I focused on recalling at least one or two home remedies of each condition and began instructing patients accordingly. I found it not only helped me give patients more than drugs, but it also helped remind me that there were many factors involved in a given illness. I began to look at their fitness and dietary health along with more obvious interconnections. After some gentle instruction, patients became active participants in their care. They quickly realized they had the power to improve their condition.

If only minor directions are given at the end of the encounter, simple verbal instructions might be all that's necessary. If greater instruction is needed or other barriers are present, don't be afraid to write notes down that they can take with them. This is especially important when dealing in complex issues. In one clinic I was in, it was not uncommon for our diabetic patients to go home with a full sheet of directions to consider. They usually were written as bullet statements while being discussed so as not to forget something.

- *Recommend starting 325 mg aspirin—one a day for heart protection.*
- *Avoid bad carbohydrate choices—white bread, white rice, potatoes, pasta, etc.*

- *Keep more with good carbohydrate choices—high fiber, whole wheat, whole grain, nuts, etc.*
- *Continue good water hydration—at least 64 ounces a day.*
- *Be sure to test blood sugars at least one to two times per day.*
- *Fasting in am (before breakfast) and/or two hours after your largest meal.*
- *Can also test whenever feeling abnormal.*
- *Write results in logbook!*
- *Recommend routine diabetic eye examination annually.*
- *Continue activity—at least 30 minutes per day, three times a week.*
- *Get fasting blood work in three months and follow-up one to two weeks after for lab and meter review.*

Depending on the amount of instructions given, they can usually be written fairly quickly and are immensely appreciated. Patients not only feel more empowered with written directions, but also receive a task list to focus on before the next appointment. If the instructions are long, a copy can also be made and placed in their chart for later reference. Regardless of notes given, some sort of follow-up plan should be mentioned in the chart and conferred to the patient so all understand. *Patient to follow-up after labs in 3 months," "Patient to follow-up in 5-7 days if not improved (or sooner prn),"* or just *"Patient to follow-up prn,"* if no specific follow-up is needed. Whatever the plan, both the provider and the patient should be aware.

If, for some reason, you're unable to explain things in a way the patient can understand, have a member of your staff knowledgeable in the patient's condition try to explain. But allow them to return if your expertise is required. Remember, though it might be a problem for your schedule, it's the patient who has to live with the problem. Try to remain open to their needs.

Chapter Three

The Gentle Art of Reaching Out

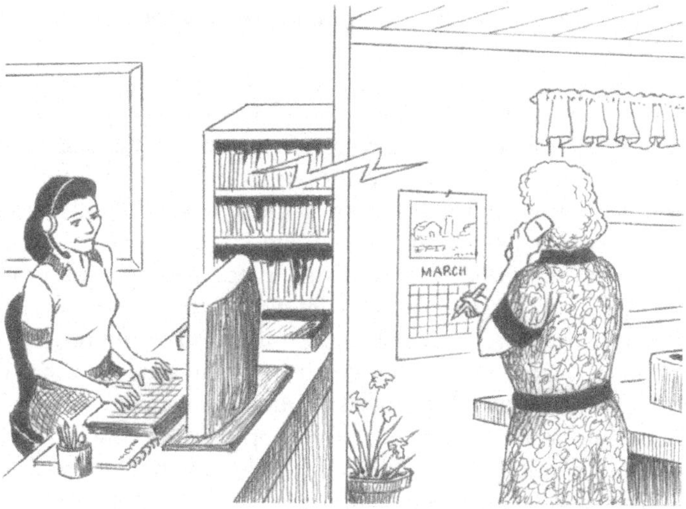

I still remember a time when phones used to be attached to walls in homes and businesses. If you were out and needed to make a call, a pay phone was usually available right around the corner. Now, since the creation of the cellular phone, talk, though not cheap, appears abundant. Gone are the days of acknowledging folks in public places. Stand in a line and chances are one or two folks around you will be on a mobile phone. Walk in a grocery store and at least three or four aisles will also have someone using one. Elevators? Subways? You bet. They're used there as well.

Perhaps it's the familiarity of telephone communication that breeds contempt. Maybe it's just not taught as religiously in schools as it once was. Or is the fact we're constantly bombarded with can't-take-no-for-an-answer type telephone solicitors to blame for our lack of refinement? For whatever reason, telephone etiquette is fast becoming a dying art. This is also readily apparent in the medical field.

The very first contact patients have with a given clinic is usually through the telephone. They quickly form opinions about the staff based on how they're treated over the phone. "She seemed subversive. She didn't readily identify herself." "He was chewing something while he spoke to me. Doesn't that doctor know how to train his staff?" "That's the third time this month they had to reschedule my appointment. They didn't even care that this is a major disruption in my schedule. What a bunch of disorganized folks."

So as a healthcare provider, how presentable are you over the phone? Well, that can be answered in several ways. Easiest of all is to take a moment and listen to your staff. As you work near them, hear how they interact over the phone. Pay attention to glaring errors such as chewing while speaking or being short with a patient. Another way to tell is to directly question patients. This can be done informally during the visit or as part of a patient questionnaire card. Something simple might get your point across like, "Were your concerns addressed appropriately and courteously over the phone?" Questionnaires, however, can be a two-edged sword and annoy people, especially if *required* at each visit. But if visibly placed for voluntary use in the waiting area, they tend to be more readily accepted by patients.

Regardless of where you reference, there are several common sense rules for telephone etiquette. First of all, ***remove all food or chewing gum prior to taking or making a call.*** A common teaching in earlier years has always been to never talk with your mouth full. That still holds true today. Speaking in person or on the phone with food in your mouth is considered very rude. It shows little concern for the information you are conveying and for the person receiving it. Emptying your mouth helps others better understand you.

Secondly, ***answer the telephone no later than the second or third ring.*** The customer should always feel important in any organization. In spite of the fact that most clinics operate in a busy environment, our society is one of microwaves and instant messages. We have become an impatient people. Not answering promptly makes the caller feel unwanted.

Speak with a smile. Smiles are conveyed not only in sight but in sound. If you smile while you're talking on the telephone, your tone becomes more pleasant. It also inspires the caller to reciprocate. You tend to think more pleasantly as well and are less apt to become aggressive.

Control the speed of your conversation. Conversations over the telephone are different from those in person. The visual cues often taken for granted, such as facial expressions and the ability to assess lip movements with sounds expressed, are absent during a telephone call. Fast talkers should be cognizant of this and slow down their conversational pace when on the telephone. This will help their caller understand the conversation better. This is especially true during repetitive portions of the conversation, such as the greeting. For instance, if you had to answer every call with, "County Waste Management and Disposal. Mr. Wilson. May I help you?" That phrase would get faster and faster each time you use it. Eventually, you risk saying it so fast that it becomes unintelligible. If your words are worth saying, then they're worth saying well.

Also, if you usually speak loudly or very soft, try to control the volume of your voice. Speak clearly and distinctly into the receiver in a pleasant manner and volume. Mumbling is a sure-fire way to upset your listener. Don't bury the receiver in your shoulder or neck. Be clear and articulate.

Identify yourself at the start of the conversation. When you answer a call, it's customary to identify the organization and your name if your telephone is a primary incoming line. "ACME Retail, This is Janet. How may I help you?" This tells the caller who you are and the company they're calling. It's a pleasant way to initiate a conversation. If your phone is not a primary incoming line, identifying yourself is usually sufficient to initiate the conversation. "This is Dr. Washington. How may I help you?", or just, "Dr. Washington."

In our infomercial-barraged world, I have seen some companies take advantage of this portion of a call and create an advertisement opportunity. "ACME Retail, where quality is king and discounts

Rx Telephone Etiquette

Answer no later than the 3rd ring.
Speak with a smile.
Control the speed of your conversation.
Let your caller know who you are from the start.
Remove all food or chewing gum.
Avoid distractions around you.
Be ready to take vital information down.
Always be polite.
When making a call, identify yourself promptly.
Ensure all issues have been addressed before hanging up.

are plenty. This is Janet. How may I help you?" Though this might seem benignly amusing on the surface, it really speaks poorly for a company. Since the company chooses to cheapen the quality of the conversation, what's expressed to the caller is that they're speaking to a cheap company. This feeling is exponentially increased with the frequency of calls made. So those who do the most business with the company feel the most annoyed.

In business, some words and phrases should be avoided. "Yeah" is a poor form of the reply "yes" and an unacceptable substitution for "May I help you?" It conveys ignorance on the part of the speaker and the company. Other avoidable phrases include "uh huh," "wanna," and "Whadaya want?" Profanities are definite no-no's along with most slang terms such as "narly" or "radical." You should also refrain from using the word "like" frequently in conversation as a pause in thought. "He's like not in right now. Like you wanna like leave a message for him?" Another habit to avoid is ending each sentence as if it were a question. It not only exemplifies inadequate command of the English language, but it can hide a true question and fatigue a listener. "Dr. Silverton is out right now? I don't expect her back for a while? Would you like to leave her a message? I'm sure she'll be happy to call you back when she gets in?"

Avoid distractions around you. Focus on your caller. It's very easy for a caller to tell if you're listening to them or if you're dividing your attention between several distractions. Until you need to use it for your caller, turn away from your computer monitor. Also, don't try to carry on external conversations while on the telephone. If something or someone requires your attention while you're on the phone, excuse yourself to the caller, place them on hold, and address the distraction. Then, when you return to the caller, be sure to apologize for the interruption before resuming the conversation.

Have writing utensils and paper available near your telephone. Often you will receive information from a caller you'll need to write down. Having the proper utensils at hand allows for a smooth transition of information and conveys efficiency to the caller. If your phone is the primary incoming line to the office, there are notepads available that are preprinted with basic information such as who the call is for, the date and time, the caller's name and number, and an area to describe the reason for the call. These pads help you not only take down information quickly, but insure vital information is not missed. Also, don't forget to include your name in any notes sent to other staff members so they'll know who took the message if further information is required.

Always be polite. When you speak to someone at home, you represent yourself. But when you're on the phone at work, you represent the company. You should be kind in your demeanor and avoid taking the conversation personally. Though it's unrealistic to say emotions shouldn't be in business conversations at all, they at least should not play an overt part. Because you represent the company and not yourself, some callers are quick to openly vent their corporate frustrations onto you. They may choose to speak to you in a manner they wouldn't otherwise use when talking to a friend or relative.

The best thing to do initially is to remain calm. If you get irate or upset, angry callers usually get angrier. Maintain an even tone to your voice. Though a small minority of people enjoy a good argument, most desire resolution. That's the goal you should strive for as well; resolution where both parties come to a satisfactory conclusion.

Listen for the main problems voiced in their conversation.

Though they might be upset with how they were handled on previous interactions, their original problem usually relates to financial concerns, product malfunctions, ineffective care, or a need to clarify information. Initially look beyond the emotional part of the call and identify the overlying issue. Focus on resolving that first in a manner satisfactorily for all concerned.

Think of it in terms of a walk. You want the caller to see you standing beside them, guiding them as they travel through unfamiliar territory towards a mutually satisfying conflict paradise; "Resolution-land." Taking on the negotiating finesse of a baseball umpire and verbally "getting in their face" won't get either of you anywhere. The "umpire approach" never seeks to benefit all concerned. Instead, it puts company satisfaction above customer satisfaction. This position is a hollow win, since the end result is that customers leave dissatisfied. A company without customers eventually quits being a company.

But suppose the patient chooses to take the "raging bull" position and verbally berates you from the start of the call? Allowing them to take you down angry tangential paths doesn't benefit anyone. They need to understand that these paths are only dead-ends when seeking Resolution-land. For instance, a patient may be angry that a doctor rescheduled a clinic day. Arguing about how inconvenient it is for the appointment date to change still does not resolve the issue. Yes, the patient may need to "vent" a bit regarding the change, but then the problem needs to be addressed. It's like having the road you usually take home washed out by a mighty rainstorm. As you stand on the edge of the new river, you may complain about the inconvenience it caused, but eventually you need to start looking for another way home or a hotel for the night.

You might say to the patient that you apologize for the change and you acknowledge the difficulties it created, but which new date would be most beneficial for their new appointment? This sort of statement let's them know you hear their concerns, but it also keeps them focused on the matter at hand; rescheduling their appointment. You may even offer to note the complaint on their behalf and have the manager give them a callback later. That may further alleviate their concerns. If they persist in their dissatisfaction, consider having them speak directly to the office manager.

If you are calling someone, be sure to identify yourself to whoever answers the phone. It's common courtesy to announce yourself at the start of a call. If you are speaking for yourself, announcing your name is usually sufficient. If you are calling on behalf of a company or clinic, then you should announce who you are and who you represent. "Hi. This is Jeanette from the family practice clinic. Is Mr. Smith available?" Stating your request prior to identifying yourself forces the person answering the phone to initially guess who you are.

Ensure both parties' issues are addressed before ending the call. Once you have concluded the obvious reason for the call, be sure to ask, "Is there anything else I can help you with?" This will allow the caller to bring up any other pressing issue before completing the call. Once all concerns have been dealt with, it's customary to end a conversation with something like, "Thank you for calling," or "Have a nice day." Similar pleasantries can be used for ending a call that you've made.

These ten guidelines are basic standards for creating a positive and helpful environment over the phone. They obviously don't address every type of conflict you might encounter, but they are broad enough to provide insight and direction in almost any telephone encounter. It's important to remember that the patient begins evaluating your clinic the first moment their telephone call starts. Care should be taken to make sure all forms of interaction end on a positive note.

Chapter Four
Office Ambience

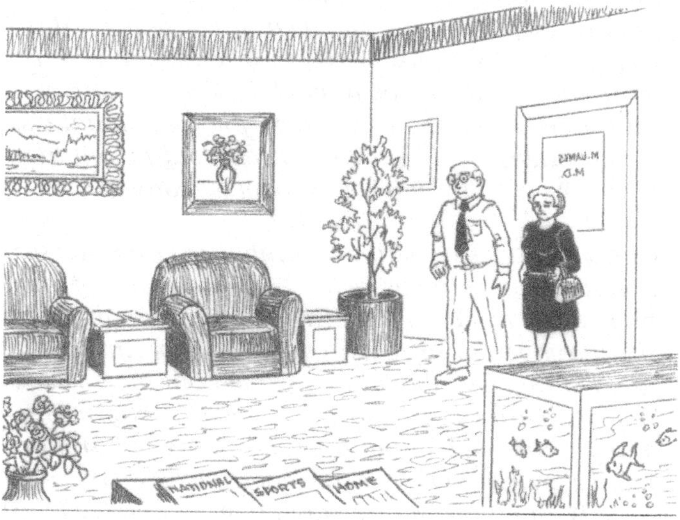

Some areas of bedside manner appear less flexible than others. Such is the case with building architecture. Early clinics were designed without significant regard for patient comfort or privacy. They mainly focused on productivity and maximizing floor space. As trends change, office layout continues to be thought of as a limiting factor in the new comfort/privacy equations. In reality, many changes are possible to improve the privacy and overall experience of the patient. Small adjustments in these areas will reap great dividends later in patient satisfaction.

The Waiting Room

Cindy L. was a 36 year old with a long history of hypertension. She had recently moved to Jacksonville, Florida and called the neighborhood family practice clinic to establish her care there. On her appointment day, she arrived 15 minutes early to fill out any neces-

sary paperwork. Upon entering the waiting room, she became a bit apprehensive. The stark white walls and outdated furnishings were reminiscent of 1970s public coin-operated laundromats. Walking up to the counter, she was greeted by several staff members engaged in conversation having to do with social activities of the previous evening or some other "pressing" issue. After a brief delay, the one nearest her asked, "May I help you?" "Yes, I have a 10:30 appointment with Dr. Johnson." She then took a quick look at her computer and stated, "Oh yes, you're here for your initial visit for hypertension. Please take a seat and fill out these forms. We'll call you when a room is ready."

Cindy looked around the waiting room and saw several seats not being used. Though one or two of them had some unidentifiable dried stain on the seat, she managed to secure a chair that appeared to be fairly stain-free. She promptly filled out the forms as requested and began to take in her surroundings. Many of the magazines were 1-2 years old and primarily focused on NASCAR; not a favored subject of hers. Without any music playing overhead, the main source of interest became the front desk. As patient's arrived, it was easy to hear their interaction just a few feet away. The young lady that arrived a few minutes behind her was seeing another doctor for an annual pap exam. The gentleman that was behind her had a rash. By the way he rubbed his pants pockets, it wasn't hard to put two-and-two together on where the rash was located.

Telephone conversations were also within easy ear-shot. Mrs. R was behind in her payments and the front desk person was informing her that until things changed, she would not be able to be seen again in the clinic. Miss K. was told her pap was normal, but because of her mammogram findings, they wanted to reschedule a follow-up in 3 months. It was around that time that a 3 year old boy and his mom entered the waiting room.

He wasn't well attended, but the office staff seemed oblivious to the happenings beyond their desks. That, coupled with the fact that Cindy had been waiting over an hour without any hope in sight made her decide to cancel her appointment and seek care elsewhere.

The first personal encounter the patient has with the clinic is in the waiting room. As with any house or building entered, all senses are alert for new inputs and are quick to make their reports. The eyes gaze throughout the room looking at color schemes and pattern changes. The nose senses variations in blended scents. Every footstep announces an arrival, be it soft or hard. Auditory interactions are discovered quickly and alert the patient to areas of activity.

Sight

Addressing the senses individually, let's begin with the eyes. When you open the door to the waiting room, look to see what greets you first. Some clinics start with the receptionist's desk at the door. Others open into the waiting room. Regardless, it should feel inviting. What about the floor coverings? Are they comfortable to walk or stand on and do they enhance the overall room environment? Can patients with wheelchairs and walkers get around easily without being hampered? Do they help improve the noise level of the room?

Color also helps to enhance a room. White, though a symbol of innocence and purity, has never been considered an inviting color and many clinics shy away from using it on their walls. Yellow is also infrequently used since people are angrier and babies cry more in yellow rooms. Green is known as a calming color and is very popular in a waiting room environment. Blue is also thought to be a sign of tranquility and tends to have peaceful results with patients. Red, a color of attention, tends to excite the viewer and is often the color of choice in sports cars. Using it as a furniture color may help point people to seating locations. Brown is known to be a reliable color, implying a genuine demeanor. Pastels and earth tones tend to work better in the clinic setting. Wood molding also helps create an air of comfort and elegance.

Now let's examine the general layout. How are the chairs arranged? Those who design chair arrangements are usually unfettered by disability. Consider sitting in a wheelchair and rolling around the room. Is there enough space to do that and still allow for leg room for seated patients? Can a heavy-set person also get around the room easily? If not, then adjustments need to be made. How about the chairs facing other chairs? These patients will be "eye to eye" whenever they look up. Infringements in personal space should be kept to a minimum to improve comfort while waiting.

> *Denise was a 25 year old business professional who went to a neighborhood clinic complaining of urinary frequency. Upon her arrival to the clinic, she was instructed to go to the bathroom at the opposite end of the waiting room and provide a urine sample for evaluation. Once inside, she noticed that the only cups present were small paper cups and no writing utensils to identify the owner. After working hard to get urine into the cup without overfilling or splashing, she felt somewhat embarrassed having to carry the uncovered sample through the entire waiting room and present it to the receptionist. The sample remained on the desk throughout the entire time she waited for her appointment. Not willing to repeat the event, she made a mental note to use another clinic in the future.*

Facilities should be user-friendly. If specimens are required while in the waiting room, they should be easy for the patient to label, acquire, and transport without drawing undo attention. If that can't be achieved, then consider getting all specimens after the patient has been taken into the back.

Can the back areas of the clinic be seen from the waiting room? If people in patient gowns or other forms of undress travel in the back hallways, are they visible to those who are waiting? If any exam doors are open, can visitors see into them from the front area? If so, consider hallway doors or other barriers to help maintain privacy.

A focal centerpiece is another consideration for amusement and enjoyment. This concept can be seen throughout the community. Restaurants often use aquariums or large terrariums as focal points of visual creativity. Shopping malls often change their focal centerpieces to include not only terrariums, but intricate wood or metal sculptures and play areas for children. Even televisions, whether by themselves or incorporated into some other visual landscape, are used ubiquitously to entertain guests. Whatever centerpiece is considered, it's nice to give patients something to focus on instead of just the other patients.

The type of patients visiting should also be considered when selecting a centerpiece. For example, placing a waterfall display in a urology clinic might not be the best idea for creating a relaxing environment for patients suffering from overactive bladders, urinary tract infections, or retention. Or live plants in an allergy clinic may pose a risk as well.

Another concern is reading material. For many clinics, this becomes an important part of the waiting room experience. It's one of the primary visual distractors that are cheaply available to waiting patrons. Yet some clinics pay very little attention to them. Often magazines are allowed to sit on waiting room tables for months beyond their initial printing. Other clinics present a limited list to their patients. Instead of a broad selection of interesting topics to all genders, they only consider the female or male patients. This is more commonly the case in specialty clinics. Pediatrics, for example, might have more female related reading material in the belief that moms take the patient to the clinic and not dads. Though this might be true a majority of the time, it obviously is not always the case. Also, some moms like reading about things socially considered male subjects, such as sports. Addressing as many different desires as possible in the selections available will be well appreciated.

Some clinics don't even think about the reading material they have in their waiting room and instead place out anything that comes into the clinic from their staff. Though it's possible to acquire an eclectic range of magazines this way, it also increases the risk of presenting something less desirable on accident. One waiting room I visited had magazines devoted to leisure time for physicians on display. Considering my appointment time was delayed and I was expecting to pay a significant amount for the visit, the magazine seemed more of a slap in the face and had an adverse effect on my mood prior to meeting the doctor.

Sound

With eyes closed, sound becomes the next most common attention-getter. And the squeaky wheel gets the attention first. In a clinic waiting room, the loudest area is usually the front desk. Here, private information is given in preparation for the visit. If the remaining area is relatively quiet, the front desk "entertainment value" increases significantly. For the naturally curious, there's nothing more inviting than to be within ear-shot of a private conversation and hear intimate details without effort. This can be especially concerning in sensitive specialties such as urology or gynecology. There should be a way for a patient to describe their personal information and chief complaint without other patients listening in.

> *Peggy arrived at the radiology clinic early for her routine mammogram. The waiting area was small and it appeared that things were moving slowly. Not a seat was available and all the reading material seemed in use. People were looking around as if seeking anything of interest to pass the time. After acquiring her name, the front office clerk pulled up her information on a computer and started verifying her information out loud. "No change to your address or phone number?" "That's correct." "You're not taking any new medication or have any new drug allergies?" "Correct." "And you have breast implants?" Peggy felt that statement echo all the way across the room. She sensed all eyes boring into her back, judging her from a distance. She leaned into the receptionist and quietly but firmly stated, "I would have appreciated a bit more discretion on your part." Though no further questions were asked, the damage had already been done.*

Barriers between waiting patients and the front desk are helpful in decreasing the ability of others from hearing details of incoming customers. They also aid in disrupting the visual spectacle from waiting patrons. Depending on their design, they can even be a signature visual of the waiting area and enhance the overall ambience of the clinic. If a television is used, it can serve as a visual and audible distractor for waiting patients. An elevated shelf in front of the desk also helps muffle conversation, both live and over the phone.

Can any conversations from the back area be heard in the waiting room? No interaction from the exam rooms should be audible up front. If so, that's a serious problem that needs prompt attention. Patients who can hear other patient visit conversations quickly realize their visits are open to the general public as well. Are phone calls or hallway conversations from the back easily heard in the waiting room? They too should be indistinguishable to others.

Music piped in overhead can greatly help to block distant conversations. It should be set loud enough to hear easily, but soft enough not to obstruct nearby communication. It should also be a comfortable style for both young and old. Heavy metal, rap, and extreme versions of other types of music (such as jazz or country) might annoy most visitors quickly. Light jazz, light rock, classical, or other similar styles are usually preferred in clinic settings.

Smell

Smell is also an issue to consider. The overwhelming scents of freshly drilled dental enamel and mixed amalgams are readily apparent in any dental office waiting room. In general practice clinics, the overriding smell is usually one of cleaning products. Sometimes, less desirable olfactory offerings rise and take flight. While working in a urology clinic, it was not uncommon to have patients with urinary incontinence come for a visit. Those with chronic incontinence usually had their adult diapers on and posed less of a risk to the waiting room ambience. But for those whose incontinence was a recent addition to their list of problems, they were often less prepared and had very few barriers to protect them from discovery or collateral damage.

Regardless of the type of clinic, patients frequently bring unpopular smells into common areas. Patients with urinary or bowel incontinence, poor hygiene habits, nauseated/vomiting patients, heavy smokers, and those who work around strong chemicals or fuels can quickly alter the conditions of a room just by entering. Strong perfumes can also be as repulsive to the unprepared nostril as any other scent. Policies and plans should be in place to address such contingencies promptly, thereby diminishing their overall effect on others in proximity.

But even without any additional input from the patients, clinics themselves have inherent smells which should be identified and considered for their negative impact on others. The scent of freshly cauterized tissue or chemicals such as formalin and phenol carry a pungent aroma that many find unpleasant. Even something as palatable as freshly cooked home-made delights brought in for the staff can be disheartening to those who came to have fasting labs drawn.

Touch

Another area to address is tactile sensations. This mainly comes in the form of furniture comfort. Are the seat sizes inviting for many types of patients? Are the seat rests sufficiently comfortable to allow someone to remain in them for a substantial period of time (1-2 hours at least)? Do the arm-rests provide a relaxing position to compliment the chair features, or are they quick at putting elbows to sleep?

The Back Area

The back area of a clinic, usually seen only by escorted patients, carries the greatest risk of unintentional exposure. Folks, after changing out of their clothes, may need to get around for restroom use or to transfer to a special location for IV hydration or other treatments. Care should be taken to minimize this sort of traffic and improve patient privacy. Consider offering a sheet to help cover exposed areas, or at least having a staff member stand between the patient and open areas of the clinic.

> *Rebecca went for her annual pap exam. Her regular doctor was unavailable, so she took a chance at another clinic. They eventually got her into an exam room and asked her to undress and put on what she felt was the mini-skirt version of the paper gown. Feeling embarrassed enough waiting in the exam room, a heavy-set nurse with an ample supply of attitude came into the room an announced, "You must use the restroom before the exam." When Rebecca said she didn't feel a need to go, the nurse reiterated. "It's the clinic policy that all patients go to the restroom before any internal exam." So she was then escorted out of her room, down what seemed like a very long hallway (including one area within easy viewing of the waiting room) and into the restroom. After waiting a sufficient amount of time without results, she was then escorted back to her room to await her turn. She decided that would be her last visit there.*

Be cautious of policy that creates unnecessary activity. The above issue could have been avoided in many ways. Upon arrival, the patient could have been notified to empty their bladder if needed. That would have been done while they were still dressed and comfortable. Upon calling the patient out of the waiting room, staff might ask once again if a restroom break is needed before their exam. Once in the exam room, the patient should be allowed to remain there until redressed. Forcing a patient to void when they don't feel the need only shows poorly thought-out policy and frustrates all concerned.

If needed, bathrooms should be within easy access of the exam rooms and away from areas that are exposed to curious eyes. Windowed doors and waiting room hallways should have adequate barriers to insure patient privacy. If possible, even staff traffic should be limited in exam room areas to decrease the risk of accidental patient exposure.

> Rx WHEN PEOPLE CAN'T FIND NEGATIVES, THE POSITIVES MORE READILY SHINE.

The Exam Room

Though function usually dictates an exam room set-up, patient comfort should not be ignored. Exam tables should be properly cushioned to allow for prolonged sitting. At least one additional patient chair should be available for any guest the patient might want in the back. The size of the room should be adequate enough for handicap access. Depending on the exam required, additional guests might best be served by remaining in the waiting room until the appointment is over.

A rolling stool or other seat should also be present for the provider. Sitting conveys a more relaxed position and makes the patient feel more time was spent in the encounter. If the patient has another guest without a chair, consider having an additional chair brought in rather than giving up the provider seat. Wheeled seats are less safe for patients and standing makes patients feel a bit rushed.

Look around the room. The colors should be inviting as discussed previously. Wall decorations should enhance the atmosphere of the room, not detract. Nature scenes, cloud formations and the like are comfortable visuals. They help the patient visually escape from their present situation. Some choose to put up medically relevant posters around the room. If tastefully done and acceptable for all ages, they can be educationally worthwhile, though not often as comforting. If many patients will be examined in stirrups or supine, consider placing something visually relaxing on the ceiling above the exam table. Be sure it's something easy to see or read from a distance. This will provide a mental break for the patient during the exam.

Exam rooms that double as provider offices pose particular

challenges to patient well-being. Patients of the opposite sex should never have to undress in front of a provider or other staff member. Women, in general, should not have to undress in front of anyone, regardless of their gender. Modesty should be considered with all patients. Have appropriate paper or cloth gowns readily available and be sure to briefly explain their use, "Just get out of your clothes and put this gown on like so…with the open end in the back. Then have a seat on the table and I'll be back shortly." Showing them where their arms go is very helpful since folded, many of these gowns look nothing like familiar clothing. By explaining things up front, you get a happier, less-confused patient.

The best course of action is to leave the room while the patient undresses. If you feel you must stay in the room, two things should happen; a curtain should be between you and the patient and a chaperone should remain in the room the entire time the patient is undressing. This protects both you and the patient from risk.

If possible, place most of the working supplies in drawers so they're out of immediate view. Speculums and other instruments (especially viewed over time, such as while waiting for you to arrive) tend to make some anxious. Keeping patients in a comfortable zone will do wonders for their overall well-being. Biohazard waste bins should also be hidden until needed. Sharps boxes not only look bad on a counter, but they inspire theft in those who desire needles and syringes.

Music in the exam rooms should be avoided. Patients often get large quantities of valuable information during a visit. Exam rooms need to be quiet to help improve understanding. Music only acts as interruption for both the patient and the provider.

By addressing style and flow of the office, simple distractors can be avoided. When people can't find negatives, the positives more readily shine. Only then can the staff and providers hope to succeed in creating a pleasant experience overall for the patient.

Chapter Five
How To Handle Specific Types Of Patients

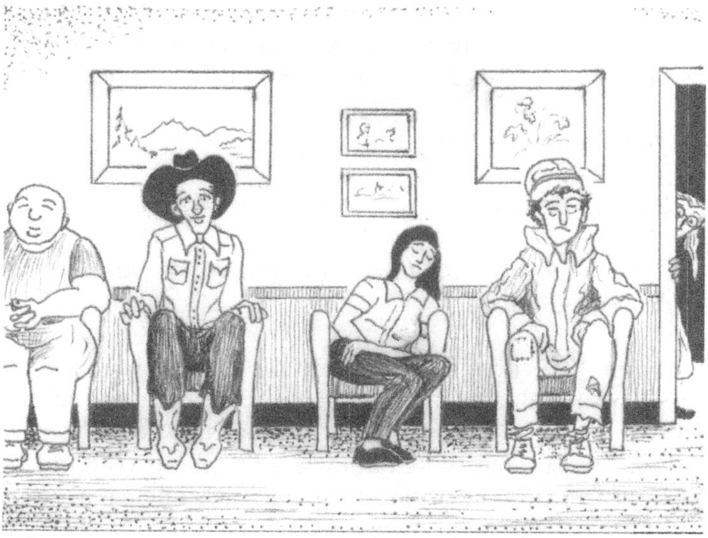

Many years ago, there was a television show called *Let's Make A Deal.* Contestants were awarded various gifts and then the host would give them choices. "You can keep the $200 in your hands, or exchange it for what's behind door number 3." The unknown behind door number 3 could be anything from a new car to a hard-boiled egg.

For the healthcare provider, patient care acts much the same way. You never know what awaits you behind the next door. The only clue is usually what's written down as the chief complaint in the chart. Even catching a glimpse of the patient in advance holds no guarantees. Some of the nicest people I ever met looked a bit unusual and some of the sweetest looking ladies I thought would be a joy to treat had hearts of stone and demanded much. You truly can't judge a book by its cover.

It would be wonderful to be able to totally trust you patients' statements and actions. But that would just be naïve. Patients often come with motives and hidden agendas. Part of being a good clinician is seeing beyond the obvious and finding the real issues beneath. Sometimes those issues are personal gain, as with the drug seeker. Sometimes they're there to hide something, as with the abused.

I learned a very cynical list of rules while in school. Our teachers said it to us frequently to remind us to be wary.

> *All patients are liars.*
>
> *All patients are dumb as rocks.*
>
> *All women of child bearing age are pregnant until proven otherwise.*

Over time I've come to appreciate the truth behind the cynicism. To say all patients are liars is to remember that there is always more going on than just what's spoken. You need to understand what the examination is telling you and how it differs from the explanation. If inconsistencies are found, then further evaluation is needed.

> *Janice came to the ER with a bruise over her right cheek complaining of falling from her bicycle onto the sidewalk. She said she wasn't going too fast, but her wheel caught between two uneven sections of concrete and caused her to crash. She said her right shoulder and hip also was sore and she desired some pain medication for it. Looking at her facial bruise, it seemed odd since there was no skin abrasion one would expect from rubbing up against concrete. Also, the bruise was on the soft part of her cheek and not over any bony surface that would be more consistent with striking the ground. It was obvious that her injuries were related to someone striking her on the face and had nothing to do with a bicycle accident.*

To recall that all patients are dumb as rocks is to remind yourself to use simple explanations when discussing complex issues, no matter how much knowledge a patient claims to have. Expecting them to be proficient in medical knowledge would be like expecting all healthcare providers to be proficient in automotive or plumbing repair. The fact that anybody is well versed in one area of life has nothing to do with their ability to grasp medicine. It's not uncommon for patients to feign understanding so as not to appear "stupid." By taking the time to explain things, it lets the patient know you're willing to help them understand and you won't judge them for their lack of medical knowledge.

Remembering that all women of child bearing age are pregnant relates closely to the first rule. It helps to remind you to verify pregnancy status whenever the results might impact the care given. Over the years I've had many women tell me there's no possible way they could be pregnant only to revise their position in light of positive lab results.

Several patient types are common to most treatment facilities. Each type poses both new challenges and potential pitfalls for the provider. Even separated out by types, no one response is 100% effective every time. Each patient needs to be addressed individually. The following list serves merely as a guide to help focus your thoughts.

The Self-Conscious Patient

This patient holds particular risk for the staff and provider. They're usually self-conscious because of an obvious problem such as a visible skin abnormality or odor related to incontinence. The most common presentation however is obesity.

Obese people cannot hide their condition. They carry it with them wherever they go. Among other obese people, they tend to blend fairly well. But in the general population, they're forced to confront their dilemma daily. Adjustments for large individuals are rarely made easily in restaurants and shops. Though subjecting someone with cancer to ridicule would seem unconscionable, people openly scorn the obese without a second thought.

Unfortunately, this behavior often carries through into the clinic setting. If not thought about when originally planned, the waiting room may not adequately accommodate such folks. If forced to stand, they only become more obvious to those around them. Once in the back, they're required to weigh in. This activity commonly elicits at least a "holy cow" or a "wow" from some thoughtless staff member. If the scales can't handle the weight requirements, alternatives must be considered. And once in the exam rooms they might have to undress, thereby removing the last sense of security between them and the outside world.

Coping mechanisms abound in such patients. They're either the "jolly" type that turn everything into a joke to help distract from the issue, or they're the forceful personality who's use to "throwing their weight around." In their own environment, they're comfortable and feel fairly protected. But in a clinical setting where health is not only discussed but evaluated, coping mechanisms tend to strain. Patients sometimes become timid in an attempt to diminish their target area.

For the healthcare provider, it's easy to focus purely on the condition and lose sight of the patient totally. Though cloaked in the guise of patient care, we become as hurtful as the school bully. "Well, you just need to lose weight..." "You're obviously eating way too much..." "I'm sorry, but I can't help you until you get this weight off."

If specific help is requested, don't give general answers. "Doctor, how can I lose some weight? What should I do?"

"Well, just get out and exercise more. And also start dieting."

Many obese patients describe that scenario as a very common interaction with providers. Even when efforts are being made to improve, providers still default to pat answers. "I've been trying to get out more. I'm walking in my neighborhood and gardening more."

"Well, you're obviously not doing enough. You need to do more dieting and exercise because you're just too fat."

One of the urologists I worked with told me why he was willing to perform incontinence surgery on obese patients. "Dave, these obese folks have been abused by many docs in the past. They came hoping for help and all they got was 'You're too fat. Lose weight.' Think about it. If that were the whole issue, all fat people would be incontinent. But that's just not the case. Fat people deserve to be continent, too. Yes, we try to point them in a healthy direction, but we also try to correct their present problem now and improve their quality of life."

As providers, we must strive to inspire compliance in our patients, not force them into submission. I always seek opportunities to praise the patient, thereby lifting their spirits. If they require more exercise than they're getting, I praise then encourage. "That's great that you're getting out more. That kind of dedication is going to pay back in dividends! It might also help if you try and add in a bit of exercise that gives your heart some workout as well. Maybe walking or using a stationary bike or even water aerobics. Not so much that you feel like you're trying out for the Olympics, but where you feel a little winded to speak at the end. If you did that at least three times a week, I'm sure you'd start seeing more results sooner."

The praise then encourage technique helps to validate their efforts and gives them a sense of accomplishment, however small. This is critical to get further buy-in on any additional requests. Once they realize you truly are acting as a friend, they're more open to suggestions.

While working with diabetics, I found many of them self-conscious about their lack of documentation before coming to see me. It would be very easy to take the bully approach and berate them for their poor performance. But timid patients are very susceptible to negativity. Instead, I would search for an avenue to present honest praise and then encourage continued vigilance. "You know, your previous A1C showed you were keeping your diabetes in much better control. That really helps to reduce your risk of complications in the future. But waiting every three months for me to tell you how you're doing only makes it that much more challenging for you to keep things in check. If you did your own finger-stick tests at least once a day, you'd be in a better position to know which direction your blood sugars were going and correct it more quickly."

Though the example showed a mild, back-handed sort of praise for past efforts, it still places the information in a more positive light for the patient, especially when said with a smile. It conveys a better message than the alternative; "You haven't been doing any self-testing at home? Are you crazy? Don't you realize that you're putting yourself at risk by not watching your diabetes more closely? If you don't care at all about your own health, why in the world do you come in here and expect me to care?"

My father used to always say to me, "Son, the best way to eat an elephant... is one bite at a time." Though a useful thought in general, I found it most applicable in medicine. Where once I saw stubborn patients very slow to change, I now see the fact that change can indeed occur in anybody if you're willing to take the time to allow it to happen. Don't expect 180 degree turns or even 90 degree turns overnight. If you can encourage a patient to just shift away from the centerline of a destructive path, they will eventually find themselves in a more productive direction. In time, small successes will breed self-inspiration and continued improvement.

The Tangential Patient

Though self-conscious patients pose some buy-in and treatment difficulties, they rarely hurt a schedule the way a tangential patient can. Tangential folks, by definition, provide information well beyond what's requested. They're quick to absorb valuable discussion time and rain havoc on a day's schedule. Keeping them pleasantly in check is paramount to avoiding time delays and upsetting other patients.

As stated previously, patients should be allowed to initially explain their chief complaint uninterrupted. Expect that to take about 2 minutes on average. If it lasts longer than that and no new information is given, consider gently assisting the conversation along.

Folks who are prone to tangents often do so because they're unaware of what's actually important to the provider. So they state as much as they can in an attempt to capture all pertinent data. Some just have a hard time thinking in terms of specifics. I once asked a 65 year old gentleman farmer if he had a fever along with his 3 days of cold symptoms. In a slow, steady tone he began; "Well, I tell yah. I just really haven't been feeling right, you know. I've been feeling weaker in the mornings than I usually do and I've just been generally uncomfortable. Kinda warm from time to time. But that might also have something to do with the way the weather's been. In my house, I have a lot of windows and when the sun is up high, it comes right into my bedroom and living room and beats right down on yah. With the additional insulation I added a few years ago, it works out pretty well for me on my heating bill. The Mrs. is very pleased. When we go to some of our friends' houses, their just not as warm as ours…" He seemed happy to continue on for as long as I would let him.

Remember, no one comes to see you with the express intent of ruining your schedule or annoying you personally. They come to receive care. They just don't have the training or communicative skills to describe their problems sufficiently. To address them in an aggressive manner does nothing to solve the issue. Some clinicians, after having endured three or four such patients in a given day, modify their patient instructions in a vain attempt to preempt further interactions. "In short and precise statements only, please tell me what bothers you today." When presented with long answers, another might say, "Please just stick to basic answers. I'd appreciate you leaving out any other irrelevant information." Basically, what those kind of statements say to a patient is, "Look, I really don't have time to listen to anything you think is important. Why don't you just shut up and let me do my job." Yes, it might indeed quiet the tangential patient, but it does nothing to inspire effective communication or confidence. You not only need to speak to a patient as you would a friend, but a friend you'd like to keep.

In tangential situations, it's better to take the "gentle directive" approach. This is somewhat akin to leading someone in a waltz. You don't yank and pull your partner into submission. Instead, you gently guide your partner in the direction they need to go. In the above fever scenario, a few interjections after the third or fourth sentence would be helpful. "Were you feeling warmer than usual? Did you actually use a thermometer to take your temperature?" If patients have a direct answer, they will usually give it up by now. If more tangents seem apparent, tie up the lose ends and redirect. "So no documented fever. How about any diarrhea or a cough?" This allows them one last chance to be direct. They'll either move on with you to the next question or will stop you and correct your assumption.

The Ignorant Patient

Even in today's society, it's not uncommon to run into people who, for one reason or another, have learning disabilities or shortcomings. An ignorant patient should never be thought of as "stupid." The two words are not synonymous. By ignorant, I mean they lack what we all might consider either "common" knowledge or the ability to process information easily. As with anybody, these individuals desire to blend in like everyone else. Often, they will not divulge such information, regardless of how obvious it seems. If someone entrusts you with such knowledge, you should treat it like gold, realizing that they're letting you in on information that makes them very vulnerable to your actions.

> *Martin, a 72 year old retired janitor, came to see me several years ago to discuss his urologic symptoms. He informed me that he only had a 4th grade education, so he didn't read very well. He was raised on a farm and had to work for the family, so he was taken out of school at an early age. He was initially hesitant to tell me because others have treated him poorly in the past, but he thought I should know so I could help him understand his condition better. Through this knowledge, I took the time to use pictures and explain some of the handouts I was giving him. I explained his med-*

ication to him in simpler terms than usual and verified his understanding. Regarding genuine praise, I let him know that I admired anyone who could take a 4th grade education and get a career retirement out of it. Finally, I made sure he had our clinic number and felt comfortable to call us if he had any concerns.

As with the self-conscious patient, the ignorant patient also benefits from a "praise and encourage" technique. It's common for society to throw roadblocks and abuses in their path. Medical personnel need to present a psychological sanctuary to all who visit. They should show flexibility with directions, as everybody is different and may need varying degrees of support. This should in no way be seen as a burden to you, but an opportunity for blessing your patient and keeping them from further difficulty with your instructions.

Inquire about their support structures. Do they have family or friends who help them regularly? Are their support structures indeed supportive? Some ignorant patients have family, but they are more hurtful than helpful. They've since grown tired of "looking after" their loved one, and often use the "short straw" mentality. "Well, it's your turn to take care of Jimmy today." Patients quickly sense this too and would rather be left confused than bother the unwilling.

Jose had been to the clinic three times prior, but it wasn't until his last visit that someone noted the patient could not read. Up until that time, he had bluffed his way through parting instructions by nodding his head and looking at any papers he was given. English was not his primary language and he did not want to appear lacking. Though Jose couldn't read a bit of English, he chose to hide his illiteracy. Spanish, his native tongue, served him no better in written form. Diagnosed with metabolic syndrome and being on several different medications, it was imperative he understood his homecare requirements. He identified one family member who could read Spanish for him and another who understood English. Preprinted handouts we sent home with him in Spanish. Handwritten instructions were given to him in simple English, since none of us spoke Spanish or could write it. Copies of both were provided so he'd have one for himself and one for his interpreter. This worked well for him and he learned how to handle his condition much better.

The above scenario shows that several issues can overlap each other. In Jose's case, he was both illiterate in Spanish and unable to speak English. This created a double problem in communicating with him. Many ignorant patients however, are willing to do whatever is necessary in order to maintain their independence. They're just limited in education or placed in an unfamiliar environment. All of us have obstacles to overcome. Some are just more obvious than others. A little extra assistance goes a long way in these types of patients to helping them remain compliant.

The Apathetic Patient

For someone who has a genuine care for others, the apathetic patient is exceptionally hard to address. In spite of their condition, they choose to ignore warning signs and recommendations. They prefer to continue their harmful activities in the false assumption that whatever their current condition, things probably won't get much worse. They often consider themselves a product of their environment and nothing they do can change that fact.

The most common type of patient in this category is usually the tobacco user. They're comfortable using tobacco products and have no desire to change. They might have even tried to quit once or twice before, but decided to continue after quitting failed to work. Many even say, "I'm planning to quit before I get cancer."

Statistics mean little to them. Pictures don't impress them. Even symptom changes fail to inspire them. I once had a gentleman come in with a 6 week cough history now producing green and brown phlegm. He told me, "I've been smoking 2 packs a day for the last twelve years and never had anything like this before. I don't think it's related to the smoking at all."

But tobacco users aren't the only examples of apathetic patients. Medicine in general tends to breed apathy through over-stimulation. Patients have a difficult time keeping up with the large volume of "must do" suggestions presented at every visit. Every specialist has his or her own requests to bring you in line with "perfect living." Go to the dentist and you'll be told, "You really need to floss more each day in order to keep your teeth healthy." For the podiatrist, its nail clipping techniques and frequent shoe changes. To the dermatologist, it's keeping out of the sun, using plenty of sunscreen daily, and always remembering to wear a hat. Regardless of the specialty, there's always something to modify or add to your day in order for you to live longer, healthier lives. It's no surprise that people begin to ignore some healthcare provider recommendations.

Where many might consider lack of action to be a consolidation of resources, a truly apathetic course must be agreed on by the medical majority, as in the case of tobacco use. And in that criteria apathy still abounds. The hypertensive patient who refuses to take their medicine and monitor their blood pressure, or the diabetic who chooses not to monitor their blood sugars or their diet all are very common examples.

For such as these, apathy will have detrimental effects over time. Changing their behavior is critical to their prolonged survival. But as is often quoted, "You can lead a horse to water, but you can't make him drink." The truth in that quote comes not from the horse being stubborn, but from the fact that you don't speak its language. Though the horse might appreciate the gesture, he sees no reason to drink above what he feels is his adequate hydration level. If you were able to speak to the horse and inform him of the long, dry journey he's about to take, he might be more obliged to imbibe.

With the apathetic patient, finding the right language becomes the task. Confrontational approaches rarely illicit a positive change in anybody. "Because I said so" never worked with our parents and should be avoided here as well. Though a few well chosen bits of medical information can help prove a point, large quantities of statistical data easily overwhelm patients and tend to nullify the impact.

Taking their apathetic stance as a personal attack also benefits no one. They need to understand that you, the clinician, are there to help guide them through their medical journey. They have sole right to their decisions. If they choose a medically unwise path, that's their right as independent people. Our job is to insure they have the information necessary to make an informed decision. As I tell many of my smoking patients, "I'd be more forceful about it if you were using my lungs. But since you're not, I just want to make sure you understand your risks."

Many apathetic patients don't appreciate the results of their actions. They have a hard time understanding how an activity they've been doing for years without apparent overt injury will someday have grave consequences later. Overcoming that hurdle can help promote change. I often tell people, "As an independent entity, you can make any decision you want, so long as you're willing to live with the repercussions of that decision. Taken to an extreme example, if you desire to rob a bank, that's okay. But don't be surprised when the police come after you, people start shooting at you, you have to always be on the run and looking over your shoulder, you lose your freedom and go to jail, your name is vilified in the community, and you lose your property. All of those are consequences of your initial decision to rob a bank."

Medicine is no different. For some tobacco users I've said, "Now when somebody later down the road finds cancer in you, whether it be lung or bladder, kidney cancer, or any one of the many other cancers associated with smoking; I don't want you to cry or pout. I want you to ball up your fist like you just won the lottery and say, 'Yes! I've achieved my goal!' Because by smoking, that's your goal." If you can help them better understand their statistical destiny, you just might illicit change sooner.

Approaching them from a non-judgmental perspective helps keep the lines of communication going. They should know that your recommendations are not based on any bias against them, but on a genuine desire to give them good medical direction and support. Make them aware that their decisions are not without repercussions. "Though what you're doing is detrimental to your overall health, I'll still continue to treat you. Just realize that as time goes on, the treatment results might become less and less effective." Or if they truly are engaged in significantly hazardous activities, I might say, "You know, because of your current actions, I really don't see how anything we're doing is providing you any benefit at all. Seeing how you're not listening to any of my recommendations and you appear to be on a fast tract to illness and demise, why not just cancel any other planned visits. It will save you some money and me a great deal of frustration. I'll just note here that you understand the gravity of your actions and will consider returning when interested in change." Said matter-of-factly and without malice, it can be very effective in inspiring a reaction.

The Demanding Patient

Patients frequently make demands upon us, both realistic and unrealistic. Sometimes it's due to their personality. Sometimes it's secondary to their frustrations either with the medical system or life in general. Occasionally, it's because they're using their attitude as a cover for other interests, as with the drug-seeker. They tend to view the provider as a medical "Genie in a bottle" who's required to grant them the wishes they desire. We no longer have cognitive input into their health. We're merely there to allow them access to drugs they feel should already be over-the-counter and within their grasp. They've seen all of the ER shows and even some of the real-life medical dramas, so they feel their knowledge is on an even par with ours. What we have to say holds no educational value to them. It's merely our opinion vs. theirs'.

Demanding patients require a calm, direct approach. Getting angry at them only gives them targets to attack. It pays to remember that this is not an opinion game. They are on your turf. You control the prescription pad and have final say (and

> BEDSIDE MANNER DOES NOT MEAN YOU ALWAYS GIVE FOLKS WHAT THEY WANT. IT MEANS YOU ALWAYS TREAT THEM WITH RESPECT AND COMPASSION, EVEN WHEN SAYING NO.

responsibility) in your actions. That being said, there's no need to become emotionally involved in their actions.

Borrowing a phrase from the Reagan era, take the "just say no" approach.

"Look, all I need is some antibiotics, okay?" "No. I really need to get a chest x-ray and lab work on you first. You might feel like you need antibiotics, but there's nothing I've found so far to substantiate that. This will help me better identify your condition and the proper medication to combat it. Without the extra tests, all I can recommend at this time is symptom relief meds."

By saying "no' and then clarifying why a different course of action is warranted, you allow the patient to share in understanding the need for change. It may not get them on your side, but at least they'll understand the reasons for your actions. In the case of the drug seeker, it lets them know that access from your end is closed.

"No. I'm sorry, but since I have no long-term relationship with you, I'm uncomfortable filling any narcotic medication today without a more complete medical record in front of me. Who was your last doctor and which pharmacy do you get your medication from? I'll have my staff get your old records from there." Some may choose to storm out of the office, but if they do it's without your prescription. Those who really need the medication will usually stay and comply with directions. Bedside manner does not mean you always give folks what they want. It means you always treat them with respect and compassion, even when saying no.

The 3rd Person Support

This situation occurs when the patient, for one reason or another, is unable or unwilling to speak for themselves. The most common human presentation (excluding the vet clinic, in other words) is in pediatrics where the patient is a child and you must deal with the parent. Though less necessary as the child gets older, the scenario might still play out in full depending on the demands of the 3rd party. Even in adult situations, a 3rd party might be actively involved either due to incapacitation or the submissive attitude of the patient.

Usually these individuals are very helpful in providing needed information. Occasionally, they assume to know more than they do and can unwittingly direct you down a wrong path. Sometimes they're more concerned about getting their own way than getting the proper care to the patient. Unfortunately, fear often plays a role in their actions. Being the sole historian for the patient, they're afraid they might not tell you everything you need to know, so they tell some fact and include interpretation as well. They also fear you might be one of those "mean" or "uncaring" doctors they've heard much about, so they scrutinize everything you do to insure all aspects of care were covered. If something gets left out in their minds, they move to a more demanding role. They demand more tests or different types of medication or additional opinions.

Remember, as the sole representative for the patient, they're under a lot of stress and only want what's best for the patient. They've cared about them long before you came along. Maintain an understanding attitude when dealing with them.

> *Veronica went to the emergency room after her 17 year old daughter Ginger took a bottle of antibiotics in an attempt to commit suicide. Though Ginger tried her best to please her father, he was a demanding individual who never really appreciated anything. He was often verbally abusive with everyone in the family, including his wife. Her two sisters had, earlier in their lives, also made suicide gestures. Ginger had just received a "B" on her report card and knew that her*

father would be angry. That's why she took the medication. Once her dad found out about her attempt, he became furious; ranting about how she never appreciates anything he does for her.

After having her stomach pumped, a social worker came in and evaluated her. She then came out to Veronica and said they would have to take Ginger to a facility 1 ½ hours away. Having younger children and a demanding husband at home, she asked if there was anyplace closer Ginger might be able to go for care. "Look," said the social worker. "You need to invest more time in your daughter, instead of just thinking about yourself! And if you try to take her out of here, we'll get a court order in a heartbeat!"

If you can create a win-win situation with all parties involved, consider doing so. Adding undo stress to any participant is counter-productive to the overall interaction. The above meeting could have been better addressed if the needs of the mother had been considered as well. It would have allowed her to meet more of her obligations without subjecting her to increased risk of stress and abuse from her husband. Instead, the social worker provided additional abuse by being unwilling to change. And if change was not an option, that could have been better explained.

Though the patient is your patient, the 3rd party member is someone the patient trusts and cares about and therefore requires establishing a relationship with as well. But this needs to be the secondary relationship in the room. Again, the patient is your primary relationship and should remain the focus of your activities during the appointment.

Interact with the patient as much as possible. If they can comprehend what's being said, try to direct your questions to them. If, in the case of an infant or incapacitated patient, they're unable to understand verbal communication, acquire the history from the 3rd party individual. Then, through such non-verbal cues as smiling and appropriate physical contact, establish a caring rapport with the patient during the exam. Even in the case of the unconscious patient, to ignore the opportunity to interact with them is to show an uncaring attitude to others in the room.

Regardless of the type of patient you have, always treat them properly. Be sure to listen carefully to what they say. Always speak in an understanding way. If forced to deny them an unreasonable request, do so in a respectful manner. Try not to judge those who cross your path. Treat all professionally and with the same care you would give a loved one. Then you both will leave the visit a bit wiser and healthier overall.

Chapter Six
The Bearer of Bad News

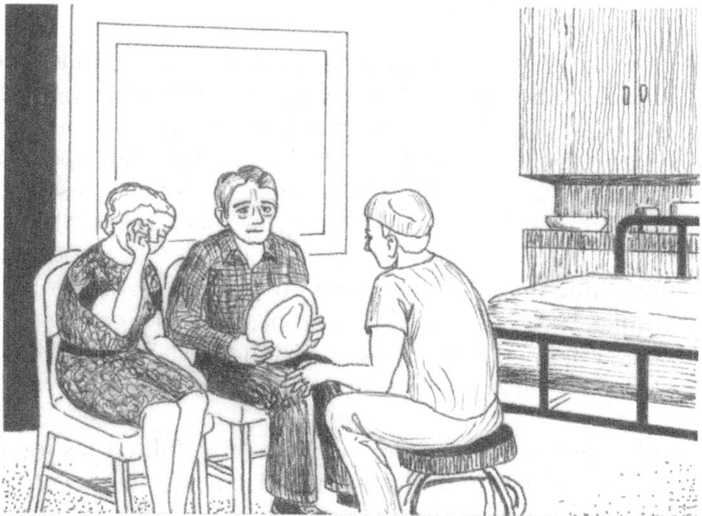

Though bedside manner has many components, the most challenging relates to one's ability to deliver difficult news in an understanding and compassionate way. Sometimes the news is stressful for both the communicator and the receiver; such as telling someone their treatment options have run out and their condition is terminal. Some news, though not life threatening, still carries great distress to the receiver nonetheless. Informing a church minister with no other vocational skills that his voice impairment is permanent would have obvious career and life changing repercussions. Informing a competitive athlete of a career modifying or career altering injury might produce the same emotions as telling the average patient they have cancer.

In many instances, it's not the information per se that makes it bad, but how that information is perceived by the patient. In JAMA 1996, Ptacek and Eberhardt defined bad news as information that "results in a cognitive, behavioral or emotional deficit in the person receiving the news that persists for some time after the news is received."[(8)] The challenge for the provider then becomes anticipating how the news will affect the patient most and the support they'll need following it. This is where the *art* of medicine emerges from under the shadow of the *science* of medicine.

Not long ago, I had a patient present to the clinic with left sided flank pain and urine color changes. She described her pain as a 10 out of a 1-10 scale and was holding onto her husband for support. Neither looked well kempt and both spoke in simple terms. While an IV was being established, I discussed her symptoms with her and made a few quick notes. She had never had urinary stones before, but that seemed the most likely working diagnosis. I casually mentioned that I would do a few quick tests because urinary stones might be causing this. The patient immediately broke down in tears and started yelling, "Oh God, please no. I don't want to have any surgery!"

Though I never even mentioned the possibility of surgery, the patient made an assumption and quickly jumped to an incorrect conclusion. I calmly informed her that no surgery was being considered at this time. All we were doing was taking some blood and urine samples and getting an x-ray. I also told her that many kidney stones pass on their own after a time of hydration, pain medication, and waiting. This information, coupled with a genuinely caring attitude, allowed her to regain her composure and accept further care. She eventually was found to have a very small stone and, much to her joy, passed it without surgical intervention.

In unfamiliar territory, it's easy to take a wrong turn. Patients are not usually well versed in medical terminology or procedure. We in the medical community need to always remain cognizant of that and strive to assist folks through the medical maze. This is not only true for our patients, but for anyone we feel less knowledgeable than ourselves.

I'm frequently amazed at medical professionals who get easily frustrated with people who lack understanding. Yet, that same person esteems their knowledge to be rare and valuable due to the length of time spent in school and the experiences they endured. If their knowledge was truly unique, you'd expect them to understand that and be willing to explain things readily to others. Instead, they expect everyone to know what they know and are quick to belittle anyone lacking such education. Though all healthcare providers appear to have the technical skills required for their jobs, many lack the compassion and verbal finesse needed to work in a manner conducive to good patient understanding and healing.

Dr. M was a urologist in Dallas who had to tell his patient, John, that his biopsy result was positive for bladder cancer. Now John was a local laborer and comfortable with his educational shortcomings. Dr. M proceeded to tell John about the biopsy and the type of cancer found. He mainly stated verbatim the information received from the pathologist. When John asked for clarification, Dr. M changed some of the wording and tried to include lay terminology. After yet another attempt at clarification failed, Dr. M finally gave up in frustration. "Look," he said. "You're obviously too stupid to understand what I'm trying to tell you. Why don't you go back to school, get an education, and then come back later and I'll explain it to you then."

Though I would love to say that the above story was created only to prove a point, unfortunately that's not the case. A quick review of patient encounters in books and/or on the internet show just how common this type of situation plays out all around the world. In the Dr. M story, there clearly was a lack of education. But it wasn't on the part of John. It was with Dr. M. Though his patient was a worker in the community and obviously able to interact daily with others, Dr. M failed to find the words or actions needed for his patient to understand the problem. In the end, he labeled the patient "stupid" and placed the blame for the communication difficulties on him. The patient then left the meeting with a cancer diagnosis, lack of information, a verbal tongue-lashing from a

> **℞ THE ABILITY TO REPAIR SHOULD NOT BE MISTAKEN FOR THE ACT OF CARING.**

"professional," and a feeling of personal inadequacy.

Resolving communication challenges is the responsibility of the one with the greatest education. He (or she) supposedly has the most complete resources at their disposal to address the task. If one approach doesn't work, others need to be attempted. If necessary, pictures might even be used to aid in understanding. Some patients prefer a little *medicalese* in the explanation, while others like as much common-speak as possible. Name-calling should never be acceptable practice! If multiple visits would help someone understand better, that should be considered as well.

Though a given diagnosis is something you commonly tell folks throughout the day, you need to remember that this could be life altering for the patient. Patients should never be viewed as one of many repetitive tasks or worse, interruptions to your day. Adequate, undivided time needs to be allotted to all patients, but especially ones receiving bad or sad news. In Rosanne Kalick's book, *Cancer Etiquette,* she relates the story of a patient waiting for over an hour to see his surgeon about his biopsy results. The surgeon finally poked his head into the exam room and announced, "You're a very sick man. You have cancer and your kidney has to be removed. You'll have to excuse me – I'm in a very important golf tournament, and I'm already late for it. Talk to you tomorrow."[(9)]

Such flippant deliveries are inexcusable and show no concern whatsoever for the recipient. The first rule of medicine, *Primum non nocere* (or First, do no harm) is usually associated with treatment actions. But in the above examples, significant harm occurred without so much as the lightest physical contact. The concept of care is not only a physical, but emotional activity. The ability to repair should not be mistaken for the act of caring.

As healthcare providers, we must remember to not only talk to our patients, but communicate with them. Though time is a very precious commodity, lack of it should not be an excuse for substandard care. If an extended visit is anticipated, appropriate time should be reserved to allow for it. The manner in which we represent ourselves, the treatment we provide, and our ability to communicate needed information helps create the overall "bedside manner" our patients feel we have. Ignoring any one component detracts from the whole.

Life has a funny way of creating behaviors that are sometimes improper. Take achievements, for instance. All throughout school we learn information and we take tests. Our grades are based upon how well we do, so we strive to be right as much as possible. If we succeed, we get the best grades in the class and move on to higher levels of learning. Our parents speak highly of us, and opportunities begin to come out of nowhere. After a while, it's easy to get caught up in it ourselves. "Oh yeah, I kicked that test in the butt!" "Who's bad? You got that right!" A chance to boast is not only desired, but in many cases encouraged.

Medicine often continues in that vein. You're taught the right questions to ask, the right exam to perform and what tests to do in order to make the correct diagnosis. You take written and oral exams and are held in very high esteem if successful. The better you become at finding the correct diagnoses, the more favored you're looked upon by staff and colleagues. Being right always gives you a good feeling of accomplishment inside.

> *While working in the ER one night, a pretty 16 year old girl came in with the history of being unable to walk after having competed in a track race. She did not fall, nor was she in any traumatic accident. Her legs just gave out after the race. She also was not complaining of any pain and by the time I got to evaluating her, the use of her legs had already begun to return.*
>
> *After examining her, I stepped out of the room and began writing my note and ordering several tests. I was*

working with an excellent ER physician and decided to solicit his thoughts regarding the girl. I had seen a patient many years ago who had similar complaints and was eventually found to have multiple sclerosis. I mentioned this as my working diagnosis. The ER doc had seen MS before and did not agree. After her labs and EKG came back normal, the local neurosurgeon was consulted and an MRI of her head and neck was performed. While waiting for the results, the ER physician again mentioned how I was probably barking up the wrong tree.

The radiologist called a short time later to say that the MS plaque was found on her cervical spine. My suspicions were correct! My ER doc was beside himself trying to determine the key to my hunch and the flaw in his thinking. It was a very tough clinical presentation and I suspected the correct answer from the start. Inside, I felt like I had just successfully completed a national board exam. I out-thought an ER physician I held in very high regard.

It was in the midst of my internal high-fives that reality hit me between the eyes. Although I did a good job that night hunting down the diagnosis, this was not a paper test or some cleverly crafted scenario. This was a living, breathing teenager with a family waiting in the exam room for some explanation of her symptoms, and I was going to have to tell them. I did a quick review of the diagnosis and prognosis of the disease, regained my composure and went in and explained everything to the family and the patient as compassionately as I could. I then set them up with a neurology follow-up and gave them time to ask any questions. As they left, they thanked me for the care I took, but inside I felt like I blew it. I was initially more focused on having the right answer and proving my skills than on what that answer meant for my patient.

Delivering bad news effectively so as not to impair the patient's ability to cope requires a little preparation and planning.[10] Several techniques have been developed over the years to assist providers in handling such difficult interactions. Regardless of your preferred method, compassion and honest empathy should be maintained throughout the entire encounter. One such technique comes from Baile and colleagues who, after an extensive review of the medical literature, created the SPIKES approach to help organize a process for breaking bad news. The mnemonic stands for Setting up, Perception, Invitation, Knowledge, Emotions, Strategy and Summary.[11]

Setting up basically means preparing the environment for effective communication. A quiet room, if possible, is key. Distractions such as cell phones, pagers, and external noises should be kept to a minimum. Invite only those who need to be there. This is usually the patient and one or two close family members. The final decision regarding attendance should be up to the patient. Allow adequate time for the meeting and subsequent questions and try to sit if at all possible. Sitting expresses a calmer, more relaxed attitude. Good eye contact is also important.

In understanding the patient's **perception** of their situation, ask something like "What do you understand about your condition?" or "Do you recall why we did these tests?" This allows for correction of misunderstandings and presents a foundation upon which to build.

It's good to get permission prior to explaining bad news to patients. This is the **Invitation** stage. Statements like "Do you mind if I inform you (and your family) of your test results?" help the patient prepare for new information and reassess if all present should be privy. Inquiring about the level of information to give, whether basic or detailed, should also be made at this time.

Helping the patient understand their condition is what the **Knowledge** portion is about. Explanations should be presented at the competency level of the patient. "Spread" is a more comfortable word than "metastasized" and simple descriptors for the organs involved serve better than any "itis"

Rx SPIKES

- Setting Up
- Perception
- Invitation
- Knowledge
- Emotions
- Strategy & Summary

or "hypertrophy." Also, never be afraid to say "I don't know." It lets the patient understand you're only willing to give information you're sure of.

Acknowledging the patient's first **emotional** response to the news is a way to help open discussion on an internal topic. "I can see you're upset by this news." is a way of acknowledging their feelings and showing empathy. Allowing for silence also helps patients process information and understand their emotions.

Strategy and summary are where you might want to formulate a plan for follow-up and summarize the previous information to help the patient understand better what was recently told them. This is beneficial in ascertaining patient comprehension regarding the information given.

In the journal *Oncology*, Mary Sawyers describes the 4Rs approach. This technique attempts to simplify the steps a bit. The mnemonic stands for relate, review, revise, and reflect.[12]

Relate means to get down to the patient's level. Come out from behind the desk, sit in a chair and try to get beside the patient. Listen intently to what the patient has to say and Empathetically respond to their concerns and questions. Use terms that are understandable to the patient.

Next, **review** the patient's history and treatments that have occurred. Discuss previous treatment goals and results achieved so far. Review any options still available for consideration.

If curative measures are no longer available, help the patient ***revise*** his or her treatment goals. Some desire to live long enough to witness a significant event, such as an upcoming wedding or graduation. Others desire to reacquaint themselves with friends and family. Resolution or reduction of pain at times becomes a main focus of treatment. Still others simply desire to die at home instead of the hospital. Whatever their concern, all attempts should be made to achieve any reasonable requests.

Finally, providers need to ***reflect*** on the changing environment of their roles when dealing with terminally ill patients. Most experience some degree of uneasiness when addressing palliative care situations. They lose their ability to take command and plow full steam ahead towards the cure. The focus needs to be on satisfying new treatment goals and not on cures or disease control.

Though no one approach works best for all concerned, each carries excellent suggestions. A compilation might be better suited to meet the needs of each patient.

BEDSIDE is a simple mnemonic to recall. It stands for Bedside preparation, Empathetic inquiry and education, Demeanor and delivery, Seek to support, Inspire realistic hope, Deal with questions honestly and compassionately, and Ensure understanding and follow-up.

BEDSIDE PREPARATION. In Bedside Preparation, focus should be given to the mental preparation and logistical concerns of the meeting. Have you had a chance to review the medical record and any special studies? Is a quick telephone consult with a specialist warranted before the encounter to explore current guidelines for therapy? Is there a quiet room available? Are there enough seats for everyone concerned (including yourself)? Are tissues and notepaper available? Did you turn off your cell phone and minimize external distractions? Has the staff been notified that you'll be indisposed for a while? Do you desire any resources in the room with you (medical record, films, etc.)?

Rx 4Rs

- Relate
- Review
- Revise
- Reflect

Once in the room, empathy and compassion should surround all of your interactions. Choose a seat (or place your seat) near the patient. Avoid getting behind a desk or behind other obstructions, such as the chart. Be sure to make good eye contact. Don't forget to look periodically at the other family members as well. Be friendly and courteous.

EMPATHETIC INQUIRY AND EDUCATION. A good way to start the meeting is to Empathetically inquire about the patient's knowledge of the situation. You might say, "Tell me what you know about your current condition?" This allows the patient to explain, in their own terms, what they think is going on with them. If the patient is new to you, as in an emergency room or urgent care environment, their answer might provide insight into their background education level and comfort with medical terms.

As you begin to educate your patient on new information, be cognizant of the speed and caliber of the information being given. People get stunned easily when terms such as "cancer" and "terminal" are directed at them. Watch them to be sure they're understanding things. Don't be afraid to periodically ask them if they understand the information or if they have any questions. Avoid statements like, "I'm sorry, I have bad news for you." You might instead say, "I wish I had better news today." It says the same thing, but in a more positive way. Other non-helpful statements include, "It could be worse…," "We all die." and "I know how you feel."

DEMEANOR AND DELIVERY. Be honest but kind. Always

treat the patient as you would want your family to be treated; with respect and dignity. Occasionally placing your hand on their shoulder or even holding their hand might be a welcome gesture. Understanding smiles can also be quite comforting when appropriate. Outright hearty laughter, however, should be reserved for another time.

Be alert also to your non-verbal cues. In the Journal of the American Board of Family Practice, Dr. Beck and colleagues reviewed 22 separate studies dealing in verbal and non-verbal communication. They found that patients respond negatively to such things as arms being crossed, backward leaning, frequent touching, and indirect body orientation. People responded more favorably to uncrossed arms and legs, arm symmetry, and head nodding of the provider.[13]

SEEK TO SUPPORT. Remain unbiased. While this patient is under your care, you need to be a supportive ally. Remember, they are more than just a condition or disease process. They all are inspired and influenced by many variables. Inquire about their support structure. Do they have local family members or close friends? Are they members of any clubs or churches that would be able to provide emotional support? Are there any community organizations they might benefit from knowing about? Are there tangible support issues that are needed, such as getting them in touch with hospice or patient assistance?

If family members are present, don't forget to be supportive to them as well. Patients rarely survive long illnesses alone. As John Donne once said, "No man is an island." Many relatives endure great personal sacrifice in order to meet the daily care requirements of sick loved ones. With so much focus on the patient, others feel unrecognized and unappreciated. Remember to thank them for the care and compassion they've shown so far.

INSPIRE REALISTIC HOPE. As healthcare providers, we strive to find resolution to problems that present. When no treatment is available and the disease is terminal, we feel defeated

Rx BEDSIDE

- Bedside preparation
- Empathetic inquiry & Education
- Demeanor & Delivery
- Seek to Support
- Inspire realistic hope
- Deal with questions honestly & compassionately
- Ensure understanding and follow-up

and often convey that to our patients. We assume that without the promise of extended life, there is no hope. When faced with such situations, it's tempting to say, "I'm sorry. There's nothing more I can do for you." That phrase should never be uttered! It's short-sighted and false.

Robert Frost reminds us that "Hope does not lie in a way out, but in a way through." If we think of our patients as nothing more than a disease process, we become blinded to further avenues of assistance. Though some may only want to hear about a cure where none is presently available, explaining ways to improve their daily symptoms might be more beneficial. In 2002, Dr. James Avery described how to impart true hope in patients. "True hopes are based on the fact that there is always more to do for the patient, even when there is nothing more to do from a medical standpoint." It's better in a bleak situation to say to the patient something like, "There is nothing more I can do to halt your cancer, but there's much I can do to control your pain and help you live each day to the fullest extent you can."[(14)]

True hope focuses the patient on realistic objectives and goals. Some patients desire to live long enough to witness a particular event, such as an upcoming graduation or marriage. Others hope for time enough to reconcile with friends and relatives. Some feel the need to reestablish spiritual and religious connections. Still others merely desire to leave the hospital setting and die with dignity among loved ones at home. As providers, such concerns should not be ignored. We should strive to help our patients achieve any realistic goals possible.

DEAL WITH QUESTIONS HONESTLY AND COMPASSIONATELY. After you've explained the situation and discussed realistic goals, ask if there are any questions they have and deal with them as truthfully and compassionately as possible. Common questions are; "How will this affect my ability to function each day?", "What can I expect as this progresses?", "Am I going to be in a lot of pain?", and "How long do I have to live?" Though not all might be asked initially, they're common concerns nonetheless and should be considered during this visit or in subsequent encounters.

Give answers you know to be true. If discussing life expectancy, it's better to be general since trying to be specific becomes an exercise in speculation. Say, "To the best of my knowledge, you have weeks instead of months (or months instead of years)." That helps the patient understand time available without appearing overly optimistic or pessimistic. If a particular answer is unknown to you, don't be afraid to say so. "I don't know, but I'll look into it and get back to you." This shows honesty in your answers and a willingness to continue supporting them.

ENSURE UNDERSTANDING AND FOLLOW-UP. After you've answered their questions, take a moment to review their diagnosis and next steps expected once they leave the meeting. This will help ensure the patient understands what was discussed and what's needed next. If you have reading material available for handout, give that to them as a home reference. Phone numbers and web site addresses for organizations related to their condition might also provide the patient with additional resources as well. Arrange for a follow-up in a relatively brief period of time to review past information and address any new concerns.

The goal of these methods is to better help you interact with your patient. The length of time acquainted with your patient, their general demeanor when accepting information, and the type of news being delivered will help you determine the best approach to use in a given situation. Keeping a methodical approach in the back of your mind and organizing your thoughts in advance will allow for more effective communication.

Chapter Seven
What Makes a Good Provider?

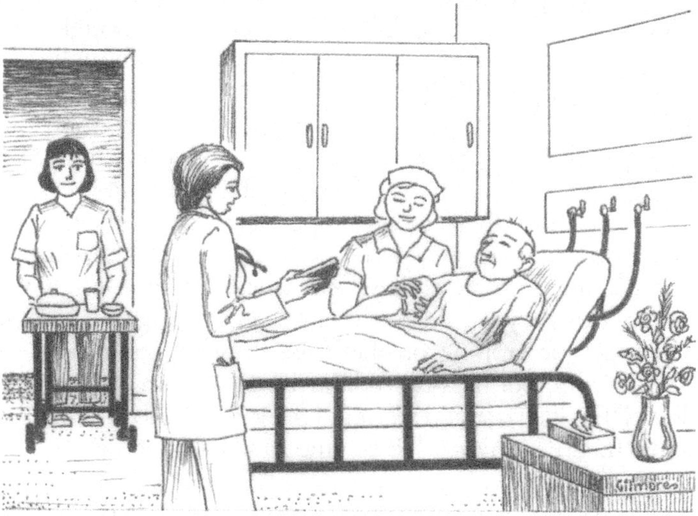

Not long ago I went shopping for a motorcycle to use as a second vehicle. It had been quite some time since I last considered taking the open road on two wheels. But the increase in gas prices inspired me anew. Each shop I entered displayed a large selection of sport bikes, dirt bikes, cruisers, and touring bikes. I quickly realized the term motorcycle meant different things to different people. Depending on your need, there was a bike to perform almost any cycling function. This variation can be seen in most anything we buy. Whether it's cars, houses, clothes, or cans of tuna. If there is a market for it, the American way dictates variety.

Healthcare providers are no exception. Whether you're looking for someone to treat your family's colds or a surgeon to remove your gallbladder. Whatever your preference, chances are if you look long enough, you'll find someone out there with the particulars you desire. Tall and handsome, blond and beautiful,

> ℞ WHEN VISITING WITH THE PATIENT, DO THEY FEEL THEY'RE THE MOST IMPORTANT THING IN YOUR LIFE AT THAT TIME? DO YOU FEEL THEY'RE THE MOST IMPORTANT ISSUE ON YOUR PLATE WHEN YOU'RE WITH THEM?

old, young, smart, witty, casual, comfortable, meticulous, or multilingual. Any trait you desire is available in each specialty, providing you search far enough and hard enough.

With so much variety out there, how do you find a good provider? Most have the standard trappings; a large office, a thriving practice, an "I love me" wall displaying their degrees and certifications. On the surface, they look similar. Perhaps if they were more like fruit they would be easier to identify. If squeezing them like oranges or rapping on them like cantaloupes produced a distinctive sound or pressure, telling the good from the bad might be less difficult. (Though I've found some willing to accept an occasional hug, none agreed to test the cantaloupe theory.)

Desiring to shine above our contemporaries, we providers begin to focus on ancillary aspects of our care. Do our clothes detract from our treatment? Is our breath or body odor a problem? Is our manner of speech difficult for our patients? Anything we can identify to correct might be the difference between having a thriving practice or a starving one.

Does giving in to our patient's requests make us good? Or can we be considered "good" even though they don't get their way? What inspires them to return to a given provider time and again? Is it purely because of clinic proximity or insurance requirements? Do they only stay with those who make them well or can we be considered "good" even when we don't cure them physically? Is it more important to be their healer or their friend? Is it possible for a "bad" person to be a good doctor? Do all good doctors have a high success rate? No one measuring tool or test seems able to objectively answer such questions. Statistics merely show what a given statistician desires you to see.

> *I was scanning a newspaper between surgical cases some time ago and read about Dr. G from Texas. He was a cardiac surgeon who had come to the attention of the media because of his high failure rate in open-heart procedures. Nothing appeared favorable in the article about him. I commented about it to the surgeons around me and a general surgeon who had once practiced in Texas actually knew him and spoke up. "You know, he's a really nice guy and a wonderful surgeon. Very talented. His failure rate isn't due to his skills or ability. It's because he's always taking on patients other surgeons refuse to see. He was often the family's last hope before giving up."*

Though Dr. G's success rate appeared poor on the surface, it failed to show the truly weak health of his patients and his compassion for their needs. If he had chosen to only take on the less serious patients like his contemporaries did, his surgical success rate would have remained very high. But those he did save prior would also have died because no one else was willing to try on their behalf.

To his patients and his peers, Dr. G was a compassionate and respected surgeon. His greatest fault appeared to be his willingness to accept patients who were otherwise unacceptable to mainstream medicine. By opening his practice to those in most serious need, he risked the statistical ridicule the newsprint eventually reported. Dr G apparently was a good doctor after all.

As for patient queries, what do they say are preferred attributes in a health care provider? Most studies evaluating patient priorities show they desire to have adequate discussion time with doctors and to be participants in their own care.[(15)] A Scotland study showed patients valued having "a doctor who listens and does not hurry me" as their first priority.[(16)] The European Task Force on Patient Evaluations of General Practice (EUROPEP), after careful review of articles addressing patient concerns in healthcare, found that patients primarily desired a doctor who was "humane." Other aspects included "competence/accuracy," "patients' involvement in decisions," and "time for care."[(17)]

The fact that most studies place a higher priority on taking time and being humane than on competence is no great surprise. It's not too hard to find people who have the general education level needed to perform in a given profession. Test taking ability and memorization, though easy enough to validate on paper, rarely measure interpersonal relationship demeanor or quantify one's depth of compassion. These less tangible traits are in much shorter supply and consequently become more highly valued.

But asking more from a healthcare provider almost becomes too much for any person to accomplish. Mastering medicine in general is like trying to catch fish with your bare hands. It's a challenge to initially grasp such a large volume of information. And once done, it changes the more it's studied. What was proper management one year becomes contra-indicated the next. Tools and medicines are constantly being developed to address diseases not previously treatable and provide new ways to treat old problems.

When the whole complexity of health care is appreciated, you quickly realize to be ordinary in ability is to be found lacking. Today's providers must be extraordinary to be considered even adequate. To be good and yet slow is to fall behind in schedule and frustrate folks with long delays. To be fast but not thorough is to risk being incomplete and possibly miss something important. The ideal provider should be fast enough to support a busy clinic schedule yet thorough enough to come to the right diagnoses. And everything needs to be served with a good helping of genuine compassion.

Dr. Mike Shooter, from the Royal College of Psychiatrists, said, "Perhaps we should be talking here of good enough doctors… All doctors are fallible. All doctors make mistakes, and we need to learn from them… We need greater support for those doctors buckling under the strain."[(18)] Perhaps that's more the case. "These bad doctors" are merely overworked clinicians "buckling under the strain."

Good doctors need to be competent enough to know what's

going on with a patient. But beyond that, they need to be able to convey information in a way that patients can relate to and understand. They also need to be able to calm fear in patients and staff and present treatment plans that are reasonable, cost-effective, and comprehendible for all concerned. Communication skills outweigh clinical competence when assessing the criteria for an effective clinician. Without it, information is never adequately transferred nor properly internalized. But more than just communication; compassionate communication is key. Though a global positioning system will verbally provide accurate information while you're driving, it's usually not referred to as "good bedside manner." That's primarily reserved for compassionate human interaction.

The type of interaction sought after today is quite different from our predecessors. They operated in an environment where their decisions were rarely questioned. Patients were expected to follow their directions to the letter. Asking for a second opinion was virtually unheard of. No one even considered requesting "options" in their care plan. Even as late as the 1970s, patients frequently felt disempowered when addressing their own healthcare concerns.(19) Communication in the clinician's office was hardly a two-way street.

Now we live in an environment of second, third, and fourth opinions and active patient participation. Regardless of our patient's education level or background, they expect us to bring them up to a knowledge base sufficient for understanding complex issues and making valued judgments about their health. Not insurmountable, but challenging in the pace and scope of modern medicine. The key to surviving these societal changes is not to look at them like a ship preparing to meet a rouge wave, but by mentally embracing them much like a surfer ready to enjoy the perfect curl.

Healthcare providers who fight such changes risk eventually "buckling under the strain." We should instead use all the resources at our disposal to assist us in caring for our patients. Our staff should strive to make all their interactions pleasant. Our office should be designed with patient comfort and peace in mind. Our clinic processes should be conducive to good flow and patient harmony. And when they finally reach our door, our demeanor and activity should only enhance the overall experience and leave them knowing they were indeed cared for by people who care about them.

> *While performing temp work for a local VA center, Dr. W met Jimmy, a homeless veteran who had metastatic bone cancer. He was being seen in urgent care because he didn't have a regular primary care provider (PCP) and he needed some pain medication. Due to the large number of veterans in the area, the waiting list for a PCP was greater than one year. Jimmy never had an easy time getting an appointment and was upset during Dr. W's visit. He acted very curt and unthankful the entire time. After reviewing his chart, she knew he needed close routine follow-up, but his condition wasn't considered service connected (allowing quicker access to care). Nonetheless, she spent most of the next day working administrative options and eventually got him on a faster track for definitive care. When asked about why she did it, she said, "I know he treated me like dirt and I'll probably never even get so much as a "thank you." But I just couldn't let him fall through the cracks like that. Not when I could do something about it."*

Dr. W. didn't just say she cared, she showed she cared. Not because of how nice her patient was or what she was going to monetarily gain from the encounter, but because the opportunity to care came to her and she took it seriously. She wanted the patient to leave better off than when he came, even at the expense of her actions remaining anonymous.

Maybe that's what it takes to be a good healthcare professional: showing genuine care for others. Not strained or contrived because it's part six in some warped 20 step caring program, but out of an honest desire to improve their situation.

Though caring is a common trait most healthcare professionals share when they select their vocation, it seems a much rarer commodity upon graduation. Perhaps the way we teach our students is partly to blame. Those with greater seniority often view junior classmen with contempt. They're quick to chastise openly because that's what their attendings do to them. The focus stays on the technical aspects of the profession, yet the demeanor of the teacher is also analyzed and absorbed just like a child watching their parent. Whether that teacher is a doctor, supervisor, or just a more senior fellow student, their actions truly speak louder than their words.

It's well known that those who have lived through domestic abuse are more likely to become abusers themselves. Yet we're quick to train our medical professionals in just such an environment because "they have to learn to stand on their own and think on their feet." "Nobody's going to coddle them when they get out into the real world." "They hate me now, but they'll understand later." "That's how I was taught. That's how they'll learn best." The science of medicine gets all the attention leaving the art of medicine to fend for itself. So in the end, to abuse in learning is to teach abuse. The seeds of poor bedside manner get planted long before the diplomas are received.

Perhaps that's where some of our focus should turn; teaching others in an environment conducive to positive learning. Not to say hiding them from the reality of failure, but allowing them to fail in a way that promotes emotional growth and understanding. They should know that poor judgment or performance is not desired and does have repercussions. But the lessons need to be handled in a non-abusive manner. Exhibiting compassion to all we meet is the best way to teach it to those around us.

Driving through Washington State, I happened to pass a billboard sign for a family practice clinic nearby. It showed a picture of baby feet with the caption, "Board certified in little piggies." That brief statement says a lot about bedside manner to the lay public. "Board certified..." tells them that the healthcare providers are competently trained to treat people appropriately. "...In little piggies" implies that the providers understand the thoughts and concerns of the average person and can relate to their conditions. It also says that they can speak the language of the lay public. Since most people notice "little piggies" after they've spent a little time with a baby, it might even suggest that the provider will take his or her time with you and not make you feel rushed.

Though obviously only an advertisement slogan, it still merits consideration for the average healthcare professional. How does your clinic/ward/office relate to patrons? Do they feel rushed in and out like cattle or are measures being taken to help them feel more relaxed? Are their feelings even a consideration at all or is the system designed purely for the benefit of the clinic staff? When visiting with the patient, do they feel they're the most important thing in your life at that time? Do *you* feel they're the most important issue on your plate when you're with them? If not, they'll quickly know it and remember. Would you be willing to take a moment and look at the "little piggies" of the baby that's with your patient?

Perhaps the system governing the healthcare is partly to blame. Is the pace of patient visits based on the provider's ability or on a generic template? If it's too fast for a given provider, it will only frustrate everyone and encourage poor healthcare. Can ancillary services and studies be ordered promptly without taking the provider away from direct patient care? Are there policies in place designed to monitor/improve/regulate patient care that only impede the provider's ability to treat efficiently? Does the staff understand their roles in patient care?

> *While working at a military hospital, a work analysis team sent around a questionnaire. It came to everyone working in the hospital; the lab technician, the front-desk person, the clinic nurse, the healthcare provider; everyone. The first question listed asked, "Who is your primary customer?" Everyone, in spite of their vocation, said "the patient." It quickly showed a serious flaw in the system. For many in that facility, the patient was really a secondary customer.*

Though everyone interacted with the patients and needed to be polite and compassionate to them, the healthcare providers were truly the primary customers for most of the hospital. They were the ones requesting the labs, x-rays and other studies being generated. They were the ones who needed the results in a timely manner in order to complete their task of treating *their* primary customer; the patient. They were also the ones that needed the system to grant them easy access and utilization so patient care was not hindered in any way. But since others thought the patient as the primary customer, they created policies and procedures that often forced providers to take extra steps and additional time to complete their tasks. This not only frustrated the providers, but slowed the healthcare process down and eventually frustrated the patients and the rest of the hospital as well.

By giving optimal support to the healthcare providers, the system in general makes care easier to accomplish. This allows providers to focus more on their patients and less on their procedural frustrations. Patients hopefully feel treated in a more comfortable environment and all staff can claim a part of the overall satisfactory bedside manner the patient experiences. With proper support, even a poor provider can shine. But without support, an outstanding provider will, for the most part, appear mediocre at best.

So what does it take to make a good provider? First of all, a good foundation is key. The computer industry has a saying, "G.I.G.O. – Garbage In Garbage Out." If you start by putting garbage into the system, no matter what additional features are added, all you'll get out at the end is garbage – with features. The same holds true in medicine. Though personal gain can be found in healthcare, that should not be the primary motivator. Someone who seeks to be a provider should start with a genuine desire to improve the well-being of others.

A good provider should be trained in and around people who earnestly care about them and their education. Medicine is a very difficult profession in itself and adding abuse in order to make the learning process harder is just counter-productive.

As with any endeavor, mistakes should be expected. But they should be addressed professionally and without malice. Discipline is a welcome necessity to any learning environment and abuse should never be considered an adequate substitute.

Finally, the support structure of the clinic, office, hospital, etc. should create policies that minimize provider interaction and allow them to focus on patient care. The more administrative activities the provider performs, the less patient care they provide. Duties that *can be* responsibly handled by other staff members *should be.* Whatever it takes to allow quality patient care time for the clinician ought to be considered.

So you see, many different components go into creating "good bedside manner." From the very first phone call interaction all the way through when the patient leaves the practice. Everything, including the policies that create the work environment, should be evaluated when trying to understand the "bedside manner" of a given facility. Not so that blame can be placed and responsibility passed, but so opportunities can be explored and self-improvement desires properly nurtured.

All healthcare professionals, whether doctors, technicians, or aides should strive to make the patient encounter as compassionate as possible. The patients are the ones on unfamiliar territory and operating under adverse conditions. Care and understanding should be palpable in all we do. And we should always treat patients the way we'd want to be treated ourselves. Good bedside manner is attainable in all of us... if we're willing to try.

References

1) Reaney P. *Doctors to get training to improve bedside manner.* Reuters London Feb 22,2002. www.cancerpage.com/cancernews/cancernews3995.htm.

2) Loviglio J. *Bedside manner test helps new doctors.* AP Philadelphia July 26,2002. www.post-gazette.com/healthscience/20020726bedside0726p2.asp.

3) Mertz MG. *What does Walt Disney know about patient satisfaction?* Fam Pract Manag 1999;6(10):33-5.

4) Connellan TK. *How little things make a big difference. Inside the Magic Kingdom – Seven Keys to Disney's Success.* Austin, TX: Bard Press, 1996.

5) Marvel MK, Epstein RM, Flowers K, Beckman HB. *Soliciting the patient's agenda; have we improved?* JAMA 1999;281:283-7.

6) Langewitz W, Denz M, Keller A, Kiss A, Ruttimann S, Wossmer B. *Spontaneous talking time at start of consultation in outpatient clinic: cohort study.* BMJ 2002;325:682-3.

7) Roter DL, Hall JA. *Doctors talking with patients/patients talking with doctors: improving communication in medical visits.* Westport, CT. Auburn House. 1993;6-8.

8) Ptacek JT, Eberhardt TL. *Breaking bad news: a review of the literature.* JAMA 1996;276:496-502.

9)Kalick, R. Cancer Etiquette: *What to say, What to do, When someone ou know or love has cancer.* Scarsdale, NY: Lion Books Publisher, 2005.

10) Fallowfield L, Jenkins V. *Communicating sad, bad, and difficult news in medicine.* Lancet 2004;363:312-19.

11) Mueller PS. *Breaking bad news to patients.* Postgraduate Medicine 2002;112(3):15-18.

12) Sawyers M. *What to say when treatment fails.* Oncology 2002;17(3):44-45.

13) Beck R, Daughtridge R, Sloane P. *Physician-Patient Communication in the Primary Care Office: A Systematic Review.* J Am Board Fam Pract;15(1):25-38. (Get the full reference.)

14) Avery JA. *Ethical Issues in the Management of Geriatric Cardiac Patients.* Am J Geriatric Cardiology 2002;11(6):413-415.

15) Albrecht GL, Fitzpatrick R, Scrimshaw RC, eds. *The handbook of social studies in health and medicine.* London:Sage, 2000:454-64.

16) Carroll L, Sullivan FM, Colledge M. *Good health care: patient and professional perspectives.* Br J Gen Pract 1998;48:1507-8.

17) Wensing M, Jung HP, Mainz J, Olsen F, Grol R. *A systematic review of the literature on patient priorities for general practice care. Part 1: Description of the research domain.* Soc Sci Med 1998;47:1573-88.

18) Shooter, M. *Students' heads are so full of lists thy have forgotten how to listen.* BMJ 2002;325:677.

19) Boston Women's Health Book Collective. *Our bodies, our selves.* New York: Simon and Schuster, 1973.